MATCHSTICK MAN

Julia Kelly studied English, Sociology and
Journalism in Dublin and worked in publishing
in London for six years. She is the award-winning
writer of *With My Lazy Eye*, which was nominated
for Book of the Decade by the Irish Book
Awards, and *The Playground*. She lives
in Dalkey, County Dublin.

MATCHSTICK MAN

The Story of a Life Lost to Alzheimers

JULIA KELLY

An Apollo Book

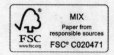

MIX
Paper from
responsible sources
FSC® C020471

Head of Zeus Ltd
First Floor East
5–8 Hardwick Street
London EC1R 4RG

WWW.HEADOFZEUS.COM

For Charlie, my mentor still

1

Now is the best place to begin. Now is what we still have and what Charlie has left. The future is nebulous; the past is dissipating, shifting, elusive, more difficult to access each day.

It is seven in the evening, three days before Christmas 2014. We are all at my sister's house in Blackrock, outside Dublin. Her small home seems to swell and sweat with our accumulated movement and noise. Potatoes are roasting in the oven, the kids are slumped with their tablets and gadgets in the sitting room, 'Silent Night' is on the radio.

I'm in the kitchen trying to sort out the fridge. It's so full that the door won't close. I've removed and rearranged things several times, taking litre bottles of Coke and 7Up from the side sections and lying them down at angles in the main part. Each time I try, the seal will stick, but seconds later it will pop open again – a dark gap where there should be light – emitting a blue-cheese reek that further weighs down the stagnant air.

I can hear the sound of our daughter's laughter as her dad tickles her in the hall. There, at least, there is a sense of space and the soothing scent of pine needles from the tree in the corner, hemmed in by a thick scattering of gifts, its branches brittle from the heat and dragged down by the weight of coloured baubles.

He says her name, 'Nipey', not the one we'd given her at birth but what he likes to call her, and the name I will use for her here. 'Do it again, Dad!' she shrieks. There's a manic edge to her small voice, as if she's almost unable to tolerate what's ahead. I picture her, eyes bright, beaming, her little limbs flailing about. I silently will her not to kick him, to try her best to stay happy and calm.

'Again! Please Dad, dus one more time.' And he tickles her again but then gets irritated by their game, her five-year-old energy too much for his sixty-five years. Her voice thins to a whine. Then the sound of her crying, Charlie's swears, the slam of the front door.

I curse, run up the stairs to the hall, give my child a careless, distracted hug that does nothing to comfort her. I open the front door and call after him.

'I can't fucking stand it! It's like a fucking drill in my head!' he shouts into the darkness as he strides down the garden path – black, angular, furious – turning left out the gate as if he knows exactly where he is going.

This morning, finally, there had been no more sleeps till her father was coming to stay. In preparation for his visit she had constructed a den using upturned chairs and blankets in our temporary bedroom. It had collapsed several times and she'd tearfully blamed me for not holding my end properly. When it was at last stable, she climbed in to try it out for herself. Perfect. This was where she and her dad would eat their ice-creams after tea.

We had been staying at my sister's since the sale of our home a month before. I had found a flat for Charlie nearby but though we saw each other every day, visits had to be kept short because he had become acutely sensitive to noise. And the noise that was least tolerable to him was that of his young daughter, whom he otherwise adored. Lately she had come up with a new way of talking to him, using grown-up hand gestures and a slow, careful way of explaining things. When she was like this he would encourage her into his arms, and she would find that familiar, warm space beneath his armpit and nuzzle in, curling her legs under her. But if she forgot this new self and became five again – giddy, excitable, silly – he would disentangle himself, get up, leave the room and lie on his bed in the dark, his hands clasped over his ears.

She had made a pictorial list of how the day of the sleepover would go and had crossed off three of the drawings on it before things had all gone wrong. We'd gone first to the playground in Blackrock Park, where we'd seen a family of swans – mother at the front, five cygnets in the middle, father at the back – waddling across the playing field in a tidy row. We'd abandoned the swings and had escorted them as they tottered back to the pond, along with an amused gathering of dog-walkers and kids. Charlie knew about animals so he took charge, gently dissuading children from getting too close. They inched down the steep slope above the pond, the cygnets sliding along on their backsides, flopped into the water and glided away, still in a perfect row.

We'd done some Christmas shopping after that – not in the city centre but in the less busy, less potentially overwhelming, village of Blackrock. I'd bought Charlie a shirt. He'd bought me a top and a Beanie Boo toy for the Nipe. Then we'd gone to a café close to my sister's for hot chocolate. There'd been a moment when Charlie wanted something on the table but somewhere between the realization and the reaching out he had forgotten what it was that he'd needed. All three of us watched his hand hover uselessly in the air. 'Mum, he wants you to hold it,' Nipey whispered, her cheeks reddening at the idea. After dinner I would run him a bath, and we'd promised our daughter that we would all go to bed at the same time, the prospect of which couldn't have been more satisfying to her.

*

I follow him down the road now, frightened, still shouting his name, still telling him angrily to calm down, but Charlie is swift and nimble on his feet: he ducks behind cars, takes sudden sharp turns, and I can't keep up with him. By the end of the road I have lost him. I want to lose him. I hate him. He is ruining our Christmas. He is damaging our child. But I also urgently need to find him, to comfort him, to know that he isn't in danger.

I run back to the house. My daughter is wedged between her cousins on the sofa in the sitting room, quiet and compliant, the way she always is when she senses that she's done something wrong. I need to tell her that it isn't her fault, that her father is very unwell; but that will have to wait till later, till I have found him and brought him home safe.

We leave her teenage cousin in charge and drive through the village, my sister at the wheel, beneath luminous snowflakes, flashing neon reindeer, laughing snowmen. We scan streets busy with shoppers – harassed, preoccupied, burdened with too many bags. None of them is Charlie, none of them even know him or us or anything about our crisis, their day is continuing as before.

Christmas no longer holds meaning for Charlie; neither does darkness or light. Or day or night, or minutes, seconds, hours. He can still read the numbers on his bedside clock, but he can't translate them into something that makes sense to him. Sometimes he will wake at three in the morning, get up, run himself a bath, get dressed and try to remember the sequence needed to make a cup of tea: kettle, water, boil, cup, tea-bag, pour. On other days he can't get to the corner of the kitchen where the kettle is. He doesn't know why; he just can't go to that corner.

We drive along residential roads behind the main street, slowing at every stranger. My sister is silent, but I know it's because she has too much to say. She is angry, partly with me for not listening – she had told me several times that the sleepover wasn't a good idea – but mostly with Charlie; never the easiest or happiest of house guests, he was now contaminating Christmas with his illness.

The longer he is gone, the more lost he will become. I think of his thinness, the light clothes he was wearing when he left – a baseball cap, his 'Fat Git' T-shirt and pair of black jeans – and I think of how agitated he'd been. Agitation was part of old Charlie, or perhaps it had only ever been part of the sick Charlie, before we both knew what was wrong. It had been months since I'd seen him like this, and I'd hoped that he'd passed through the phase, like the phases of grief, and had now moved on to acceptance, however possible acceptance is when you don't understand what's happening to your mind. The new Charlie is quiet and gentle and acutely self-aware. He sees all his mistakes, watches his forgetfulness and disorientation from a part of his brain that is still lucid and sharp and observant.

Though she is driving, it's my sister who sees him first – I've become numb and useless, as is my habit in a crisis – at a busy junction leading to the main street. She slows down, and we shadow him as he strides on, oblivious. When she can, she pulls over, and I get out. I walk towards him, tentative, call his name. He sees me and starts to run in that light-footed, relaxed style of his – the way you'd run from a child in a game of chase when you want to let them catch you – and yet it is effective. His legs are long and he is agile for his age, and I know there's no possibility of my reaching him.

He jumps a metal barrier at the lights and tumbles into heavy Christmas traffic. He stumbles to his feet again and weaves his way through beeping and swerving cars. It is like that scene from *It's a Wonderful Life* where George Bailey, drunk and in despair, staggers onto a busy road. All of this feels film-like, unreal. Someone shouts something offensive; of course, they think Charlie's drunk. He makes it across and wanders through the ungated entrance of a large park. I track him until the darkness absorbs him, throw my hands up in frustration and start to cry.

'Judge Julia' is his latest nickname for me, inspired by his favourite daytime television show. Whenever he says it, it makes him laugh. 'Brilliant,' he says to himself. He thinks I'm bossy, impatient, a 'targe', and that I'm always in a hurry to leave him.

It's true. I'm a terrible carer. I blunder in, all business, in the mornings when he's still making sense of his dreams. Today I pulled the Exelon patch from his neck while he was eating his Alpen. I encouraged his head forward, without asking or warning, tugged the collar of his dressing gown down a few inches, looked, then felt, for the old patch. His skin was still warm from sleep and the base of his neck, just above the last vertebra of his spine, looked boyish and exposed, and it made me feel ashamed of my roughness and my haste. Even so, I pulled at the old patch and it came away, leaving in its wake a circular, gummy, black residue. I tore the outer packaging of the new patch with my teeth, peeled its inner strips and slapped it onto his skin beside the site of the old one. I'd been told to vary the position slightly each day to prevent rashes and redness: the top of his back is now decorated with black circles, some of them overlapping, like smudgy Venn diagrams. At first I'd tried to rub these circles

9

away using a nailbrush, then a facecloth and soap, but it was ineffective and painful, and left his skin raw. Charlie says he quite likes them now – he calls them his tattoos.

Before I left, I made him wash his pills down with his tea, and then I moved about his small kitchen doing this and that, Charlie out of his seat and following me as I went back and forth, wanting to be useful but frightened of getting under my feet.

Back in my sister's car outside the park, I make two phone calls. The first to Charlie's ex-wife, the second to his grown-up daughter. Charlie's Angels, someone called us once. They stop whatever they were doing and tell me they're on their way. Finally, at my sister's suggestion, I phone the police. They dispatch two cars and when the first arrives, I get in. My sister goes home to check on the children and wait for news.

The policewoman beside me is chewing gum. She tries three times to mount the pavement and swears each time she fails, revving the engine and smacking the tyre against the edge. 'Say nothing,' she says to me. Once we're up, we drive along the pedestrian path in the park, and I feel briefly and inappropriately superior to be doing what no normal car is permitted to do. I watch people watching us, their greedy minds hungry for details. Another dysfunctional family, another grubby domestic, you always get them this time of year. 'Diabolical' is the word one counsellor used to describe our situation. Then he'd put his head in his hands and had said 'Jesus' again and again.

'You're in the swamp,' he'd told me as I'd paid him €150 for our session, 'and it's a very long way to the shore.'

We are still doing futile circuits of the park when the call comes through – they've found him. At first all I can see are several police officers circling something, behind a row of parked cars. We cross the road to join them and there he is, sitting on a low wall, cornered, his body slumped in surrender. He has removed his baseball cap and is holding it in his hands. *No one is laughing at you*, is what I want to say when I see him. That's what I wanted to say the other day when the doctor spoke about nursing homes. Charlie had sat listening, nodding, polite in his leather jacket and Converse high-tops. *You will always be Charlie, you will always be cool. No one is laughing at you.*

'I'm demented,' he says, staring up at one of the officers – his explanation and his apology.

'He has Alzheimer's,' I say quietly to the guard closest to me. Charlie's eyes are wild and I can see that he's been crying, but there's a playfulness in them too – he is trying his best to look crazy – and this tells me that he will, that we will, be OK.

We sit in the back of the police car together, not talking. I hold his soft, icy hand. We are dropped off where we began, at my sister's house. Every light is on, every window filled with a yellow glow, as though someone has gone from room to room in a panic. I phone her from the street – Charlie refuses to go back in – to tell her the news and ask her to let the others know.

I grip him at the elbow and guide him across the road to the Volvo he is no longer allowed to drive. He goes to open the back door, where the child's car seat is. He knows that this is wrong and with my encouragement he moves to the front passenger door, but he can't find the handle. I open it for him. When he is in and I am beside him, putting the key in the ignition, he tries to clip his seat belt into the CD holder. He has done this before and it has made him swear and kick, but tonight he says nothing, he simply holds his arms up and out of the way and waits for me to lean over and buckle him in.

2

Charlie and Skippy. I liked them before I met them; they had such likeable names. We were staying at the same artists' retreat in County Monaghan that autumn of 2004. Before we were introduced, I imagined a sun-tanned Californian travelling through Europe with his young son, or maybe a tomboyish girl. A man and his child on some sort of adventure.

I had been given a writer's residency at the Tyrone Guthrie Centre, or Annaghmakerrig, as everyone calls it, before I, or anyone else, could possibly describe me as a writer. It had been my big brother's idea – he thought it might help to get me started. I'd bored everyone about my ambition since the age of fourteen, but I was still only talking about it at thirty-five. And I needed to do anything other than remain where I was, watching the sad, ugly days of a dying relation-ship and beyond bored in a meaningless job. It was

October, my favourite month – always a time for new beginnings; the real new year for me, with its bright cold days and firelit evenings, so much more meaningful than grey and dreary January.

At Busáras in Dublin city centre, I heaved four large holdalls onto the Monaghan bus – far too much luggage for someone without a car (after several failed attempts I had yet to learn how to drive) and for only a two-week stay, and a sign in itself that my focus was more on escape and on the prospect of raucous evenings with poets, artists, dancers or musicians than on solitary writing at my desk. I would *try* to write, of course, in the time I'd been granted, but I would also be free – and who knew what might happen. Despite the earnest and ambitious tone of my application, this was how I was thinking on the two-hour journey.

I sat in the back of a taxi from Monaghan bus station, not talking. I was woozy from the stuffy bus and giddy with apprehension. What was I thinking, deciding to spend two weeks in the company of actual accomplished artists? I had written almost nothing and had only the vaguest idea of what I was going to work on while I was there. What would I do all day while everyone else was being properly creative? I was a phoney, a fraud, a salesman with an empty suitcase.

I had been underachieving all my life. I'd dropped out of university in my second year, right after my father died. College had been his idea; German the subject he'd chosen for me to study, and the only university to accept me was one he had described as the worst in Europe.

He used to roar that I'd put ten years on his life, and I'd roar back at him, slam my bedroom door, get under the covers and cry and rock from side to side to *Now That's What I Call Music 7*, forcing my voice hoarse so that boys would find its huskiness sexy.

On the night he collapsed with a massive heart attack on the kitchen floor, I'd been finishing my waitressing shift at Pizzas and Tarts café, hoovering carelessly under tables, sucking up sugar sachets and pineapple chunks. 'Where there's life, there's hope,' was my mother's mantra till they turned off his life-support machine ten days later. I was twenty-one; he was fifty-nine.

*

Just beyond the small village of Newbliss, we took a right and drove down a long, well-tended laneway to the white entrance gates of Annaghmakerrig. A putty-coloured Gothic mansion girdled by renovated stables, it looked eerie in darkness, with the lake in front of us vast, covered in a low mist and surrounded by thick forests of willows and birch.

As we crunched back and forth over the gravel with my bags, the taxi driver told me that the 'Big House' had its own ghost, a Miss Worby. What was troubling Miss Worby, he explained, was that her ashes had been scattered in the rose garden at Annaghmakerrig when she had wanted them scattered in England. Now she resided in a narrow and permanently cold room on the first landing.

'Ach, don't be worrying,' he said, leaning his head out of the window as he reversed, 'she's only interested in men.' I didn't believe in ghosts, but I wasn't thrilled at the idea of sharing a house with one either, particularly as I was already scared of other things.

*

The two women in the office were laughing about something I didn't understand. One of them was sitting in an easy chair, occasionally lowering her chin to sip from the mug she was holding; the other one couldn't stay still. She checked me in as she moved about the room, distracted, looking for this and that. Their talk was rapid, their accents strong and, though I couldn't follow what they were saying, I was smiling too, from shyness and their infectious cackles.

The busy one led me through a grand, high-ceilinged hall, where sparse Persian rugs covered stone floors and an assortment of framed portraits of long-dead dignitaries eyed us glumly. The house was very quiet and calm – it was hard to imagine that it was full. She told me all eleven bedrooms were occupied, as were the six self-catering farmyard cottages outside, as we approached the first landing.

'You're a writer, is that right?' she asked as we stopped outside Lady Guthrie's room (not Miss Worby's, thank the Lord, though hers was the next one along).

'Yes,' I replied, lied.

She held the door open, encouraging me in, presenting the room with pride. It was beautiful: large, lamplit, cream-carpeted, with a big bay window overlooking the gravelled entrance, the gardens and the lake beyond. There were a dark mahogany desk and a leather chair in front of the window, where I would work. The bed was king-sized and piled high with cushions and throws. In the centre of the room was an incongruous wrought-iron spiral staircase.

'Righty-oh, I'll leave you to it, so. Dinner's at seven, but sure, take your time. Lovely wee group we've got here at the minute.'

The first thing I did was unpack my laptop, fire it up and sit in front of it. Nothing came, of course, and I was up again in seconds and wandering around the room. I climbed the creaky winding stairs. They gave the impression of leading to something important – an attic, a gallery, a pulpit perhaps – but what was at the top was a toilet with a sloped ceiling, a tiny four-panelled window and a mirror with one of those plastic strip lights with a string pull above it. Its base was thick with dead flies, and when you pulled the string nothing happened.

Back down again, I sat on my bed and heard the door across the landing shut. Then footfalls on the stairs. I got changed and waited a few moments, not wanting to meet anyone; then I opened the door and went down myself – it was ten past seven, the perfect time to make my appearance.

I turned the door handle to see an empty sitting room and a dying fire. I retreated, stood still and listened, trying again to work out where the voices I could hear were coming from. I followed them through the hall, pushed open swing doors with nautical windows and strode down the ramp to the kitchen as loudly as I could to disguise my profound fear.

The table was candlelit and fully occupied. I registered bottles of wine, large casserole dishes, great roars of laughter. And there they all were: the dancer, the journalist, the poet who spoke only when he was drunk, the grumpy American with his pipe and flat cap, the handsome but dangerous-looking writer from Dublin, the gay comedian, and the nervy painter with her black pudding-bowl haircut and red turtleneck sweater.

I knew none of them that first night, of course; they were all still nameless and intimidating. I sat, awkward and overdressed, at the end of the table. There was no one to my left; the director of the retreat sat opposite me and an older female artist from New Mexico was on my right. Once I'd rid myself of the feeling that the director had joined us solely to check out my credentials, I settled down a little, but I talked too much and ate too fast and drank far too much red wine.

There was a brief lull when the main course was over, conversation disrupted by people standing to clear the table. I didn't know whether to stay sitting or get up to help, and I found myself with no one to talk to. I was glad of the distraction when Charlie and Skippy arrived moments later. All eyes turned to them.

They stood at the end of the table, luminescent under lamplight, the group gathering around them in stark relief, like a Renaissance painting of a biblical scene with the contrast of light and shade – *chiaroscuro*, Charlie would later teach me. Charlie was not Californian, he was not sun-kissed and not young. He was a tall and thin man from the north of Ireland, in his fifties, I guessed, entirely bald, with sunken black hollows beneath his eyes. His clothes were dark and baggy, and tucked under his arm was Skippy: not a cute boy or a tomboyish girl, but a six-foot-long iguana, looking startled and ready to attack. When he sat down to join us for dessert she crawled up his shirt, curled herself around the back of his neck and began bobbing her head. 'That means who the hell are you?' he said softly and smiled at me. He reached his hand up to stroke under the iguana's chin until her eyes began to close.

*

For the first week we were all very diligent – writing, painting, dancing, composing in the quiet of our own studios and rooms. I took a lot of early-morning walks, for exercise but also on a vague search for inspiration. Walking is a great way to get ideas, I'd read somewhere. It was often misty when I set off, the lake invisible, cobwebs spread decoratively across bushes, the air wet and thick with the delicious stench of fresh manure.

I never met anyone on these mornings, but sometimes I would catch the sound of a musical instrument being tuned, a complaining crow, distant farm machinery. Everything was in soft focus around me: beiges, browns, light greens, the dirty cream of sheep grazing on the drumlins. Ear-tagged cows stopped chewing the cud and stared at me as I passed, seeming to sense that I wasn't local and that I was wary of them. I stuck to the same route each day, walking anticlockwise around the near edge of the lake until I could go no further. I was nervous of taking a wrong turn, getting lost or encountering a hostile dog.

I ate in my room at lunchtimes, going up and down with sandwiches and cups of tea on trays several times a day, always with the unshakable feeling that I was being watched, that Sir Tyrone Guthrie was keeping a close eye on me. He had provided me with all that I could possibly require: space, silence, food, drink, a comfortable place to work – and I needed to at least look like I was using my time creatively.

But as the week wore on, our communal discipline weakened. More bottles of wine were ordered at night. We got to know each other, got giddy, started staying up late. We began to seek each other out, took tours of each other's rooms, scared ourselves with news of nocturnal visits from Miss Worby – the beautiful dancer swore the ghost had sat on her legs as she slept; the dangerous writer from Dublin said she'd curled up behind him in bed.

We saw the Northern Lights one night. Charlie still remembers them; I only remember staying up late, being outdoors and freezing, and looking up at the sky but noticing nothing except everyone else's enthusiasm.

One evening we took a boat across the lake after dinner. Charlie tried to teach me the rhythm of rowing, then stood and made the boat rock and list as he clambered over to my side and sat behind me.

He held on to the oars, his arms pressed against mine, forcing them to follow his actions. I was embarrassed by this clichéd attempt to get close – Charlie was playful and a flirt – but I liked it too. I've always liked to be taught things (I developed crushes on tennis instructors and teachers in my teens), and Charlie was becoming increasingly intriguing and attractive to me. I couldn't get the hang of the rowing – I was too self-conscious to concentrate – so he took over, and I lay back and listened to him talk. I loved the way he spoke: his soft accent, his old-fashioned (to my ear) turn of phrase.

Rowing came naturally to him. He'd grown up on the seafront in Bangor, County Down, with uninterrupted views over Belfast Lough to Whitehead on the Antrim coast. He told me stories of childhood adventures he had taken with his dog Wendy, the two of them in a little rowing boat far out in Bangor Bay, and how his mother would flash a torch across the water to let him know when he was to come home for his tea.

At the end of the first week, things changed. On Friday night we all went to McGinn's, a tiny pub in Newbliss. Annie, the landlady, was in her eighties and so small herself that all you could see was the crown of her grey head as she pottered back and forth behind the counter, her hand reaching up every so often to deliver a drink to a customer. On the wall above the bar there was a photograph of Annie when she was younger, though not much, on a motorbike in full leathers. The bar was also her home, and up in the pink-carpeted bathroom that she opened to the public were her clothes basket and nylon bath cap.

That night Charlie bought me drinks, played with my gloves, laughed at my silly observations and gave me the front seat when he drove us all home at closing time, Leonard Cohen's 'The Future' thumping on the stereo, at least six in the back – some sitting forward, some up on laps – as we careered down dark and unfamiliar country lanes. I loved that he was so wild; but also that he was the one in control. There was an impromptu party back at Charlie's cottage. I remember the dangerous writer doing a sort of pole dance around a supporting beam, some vile-tasting liqueur and then Charlie kicking everyone out except me.

We lay under a skylight and talked through the night, Skippy in the corner keeping a watchful eye on me, resentful of being usurped from her place on the pillow beside her master. Her knobbly dewlap splayed whenever I so much as moved. I had never been keen on reptiles, but I accepted and liked her immediately and I think maybe she came to feel the same. She was part of the package, part of Charlie.

There was a moment in the early morning when we were both quiet, dazed with tiredness and drink. I turned to Charlie and saw that he was staring at a shadow the rising sun was making on the ceiling. I followed his gaze and began to stare at it too. 'Hey, that's my thing to be looking at,' he said in mock annoyance. 'You find your own thing.'

I had never met anyone like Charlie, anyone who saw things the way he did. In the following days he began to linger after dinner, before returning to his cottage, and he focused his attention on me. He teased me about my tweed trousers and threadbare, scruffy black coat. I teased him about his narrow and neat goatee beard, which he charmingly referred to as his 'fanny tickler'. He said he had never met a girl with so many hang-ups; he told me often that I was a 'buck eejit' and that I needed to wise up.

He could be cruel, too. One night at a party in the living room, the reticent poet sang a Leonard Cohen song and I took up the harmony. There were a few seconds of silence after we'd finished, followed by some abrupt claps. Charlie told me later that he'd need to listen again to be sure, but that he didn't think I could sing. And he was dismissive of the work of the funny one in the red turtleneck who had a studio next to his. Every time he passed her window, he would see her arm moving swift and furious across the canvas, giving it everything. 'She's just making marks,' he said.

Charlie lied sometimes. On Monday he was fifty, by Friday he was fifty-five. And he'd snuck Skippy in when animals were forbidden, admitting only to a small lizard when confronted by the director, gradually widening his arms to take in her full six feet. She had been discovered one morning by the cleaner while hoovering, who mistook her for a crocheted toy – you could hear the screams in Carrickmacross. But Charlie's was the tidiest of all the cottages, according to that same cleaner: 'Aye, he keeps it spick and span,' she said in his and Skippy's defence.

We began to take walks together, neither of us able to focus on work. Charlie called himself 'Brown Owl' as he strode ahead of me across the fields. He would always bring a stick, years before he needed one, and twirl it like a baton in the air, or balance it on his index finger for impressive lengths of time. 'It's for getting small boys out of trees,' he said when I complained. I didn't want him to have a stick. I was already worried by how old he was, about the twenty years between us.

*

I was myopic, but Charlie saw everything. A lone donkey (or 'dunkey', as he called them) in a far-off field, the smallest bug on a leaf, a hovering, electric-blue dragonfly. As we walked, he would stop every few steps to point out the brilliance of a colour of a particular leaf, the tangled branches of an ancient tree. He gave focus to things that others ignored or trampled on or yanked from the ground. Sometimes he would come across a colour, a view, a shape he found so remarkable that he couldn't handle it. 'That's wild,' he would say. 'Fuck, that's too beautiful, it's too much.'

He could run as fast as a boy across rocks at the lake's edge, making split-second decisions on where to put his foot next. He could put a blade of grass between his thumbs and produce a sharp whistle that made dogs stop in their tracks, ears pricked; and I'd stop too and ask him to show me how to do it. He would detach brambles from my coat and my hair as we walked, free me from barbed-wire fences, tend to my splinters and cuts. I'd call him a sissy as he edged around puddles that I squelched right through, muddy water seeping into my socks. 'It's because you're Catholic,' he would say. 'Because you weren't brought up proper.' But he liked to pee outdoors, especially at night, even when there was a conventional toilet inside, which didn't seem proper to me.

'Let's use the word "literally" literally all day today,' he suggested one morning, and that's literally what we did. He put the word 'but' at the end of every sentence, a verbal tic he'd never noticed. Teasing him about it, I told him I'd heard of some children who'd been locked in a cellar for years until one managed to escape and get help. Psychologists said the single thing they had in common was that when they spoke, all their sentences ended with 'but'.

Charlie ignored my insinuation and told me about the 'Chicken Boy' instead – a child who was found doubled over in a chicken coop near Downpatrick in County Down. He couldn't stand, he clucked in hen language and flapped his arms about when excited. Charlie had caught a glimpse of him once from the window of his home on the Seacliff Road – the boy was being taken for a walk by a nurse and was scurrying about the pavement with a wild look in his eye. The image scared us both.

Some days he put 'wee' in front of everything, the way some Northerners do. It made me laugh and I'd join in. (My father would have hated his accent. 'Ah, no!' Dad would snort, unsettling himself from the armchair in which he had just got comfortable, his glass of whiskey on the coal barrel beside it, to watch the main evening news. 'Not Pigs-in-space!' he would roar, referring to a portly newsreader from the North, and he would recede, loudly pronouncing everything with a Northern accent until he had slammed his study door.)

When Charlie wanted to impress, he made me think of the mating dance of a bird of paradise – feathers out, all his best colours on show. He told me about the music video he had made for Bob Dylan that got him a Grammy nomination, and how he had worked with Bette Midler and Bruce Springsteen. He quoted from Shelley, Keats, Dylan Thomas, Rimbaud. He introduced me to country music, played John Prine, Lucinda Williams and Woody Guthrie on the stereo at his cottage. And he sat with great hardback books he had brought with him to the retreat and talked me through paintings by Botero and Don Bachardy, carefully turning the pages as we studied them together: Botero's soft fat women, Bachardy's perfect sketches of men.

He gave me a tour of his studio at the retreat, which made me nervous – I didn't know one thing about art. I remember a painting of a single red brick with a red background. When he asked what I thought, I had pouted, inwardly searching for adjectives. 'It looks angry,' I said. He flicked his thumb at my bottom lip and said, 'Ach, you're a wee bat.'

But Charlie also loved *Coronation Street* and *Viz* and rhubarb-and-custard sweets. He told me about the pulley system he'd constructed in his bedroom when he was a boy, with a bucket at the window end, and how his mother would fill it with treats at night. After lights out he would lower it by pulling the strings and have midnight feasts on his own in the dark.

We talked about writing. He told me to write using all my senses, not just sight. What did the thing smell like? What did it feel like? When you touched it, what was its texture? What sounds did you hear? Back in my room I would try to think about what he'd taught me and would sit at my desk, laptop open, hands poised. The seven senses: sight, smell, taste, hearing, touch, vestibular (movement), proprioception (body awareness) – I had to look the last two up, but I would use them all in my work. This was what I would do, beginning tomorrow.

'Go ahead, just make a mess,' the artist from New Mexico suggested when I told her that I was stuck. This I could do, I'd been making a mess for years. I'd been rudderless for so long, losing jobs, going out with the wrong men, spending money I didn't have on things I didn't need, just generally mucking things up. I didn't know it then but I was missing my dad, who had died before I'd had the chance to do anything to impress him, before I had told him that I loved him. Charlie was someone new but older, who could teach me things, someone who might become proud of me.

On Charlie's last day at Annaghmakerrig, we tried to complete the crossword together at the kitchen table. He wasn't concentrating on the words, he was doodling as he always did. Funny, sweating *Viz*-inspired men peeped out from behind the puzzle as if they were up to no good, or hid from the heavy-set, scowling, huge-breasted women in slippers he created in any free space. We both remember that our little fingers touched as he drew and I scribbled words.

*

'Did you know that a swan could break your arm?' I told him as we stood at the boathouse by the lake watching them, just before he left. It made him laugh. It still does, I've never understood why.

He wanted me to travel back to Dublin with him; I said I needed to stay. I had to see out the last three days of my residency. If I was going to be a writer, I would have to begin to take myself seriously. I also couldn't yet imagine 'us' outside of Annaghmakerrig. Charlie and me together seemed wildly incongruous, and we both had relationships on the point of dissolution in Dublin. Here, real life was suspended; it was a magical time out of time. He told the funny one in the red turtleneck that he'd race her back instead. 'That's a brilliant idea!' she said.

A few days before he left I'd shown him some of what I'd been working on, and he had given it back to me that evening with whole paragraphs crossed out, question marks in the margins and arrows telling me to please turn over. On the reverse were his own words. He had given up entirely a few pages in – the rest of it too bland to be read – and had gone back to his studio. He reappeared a little later with some of his own writing. 'This is how to do it,' he said.

After we said goodbye, I sat cross-legged by the fire he'd made for me in Lady Guthrie's room and reread the writing that he'd edited. I missed him immediately; I wanted to be reminded of his voice. I began to scribble out my words till the pages were grubby and creased. I didn't know then that this was not the answer, that this was not the way to find my own voice; but at least now I was thinking like a writer.

Unlikely mentor and misguided muse – this was how Charlie and I began.

3

'An artist in his fifties, separated, with an iguana. I'm just saying it's not ideal,' a friend said, concerned, when I told her about Charlie. But I didn't care, she hadn't met him, she didn't yet know that Charlie was the most interesting, strange, funny, articulate and original person I had ever known. I was blind to anything or anyone else. I was 'literally' spellbound by him.

For three days after my return to Dublin I heard nothing from him. I had scribbled my number beside the crossword we'd been doing on the day he left, and though he was appalled by my spidery, illegible handwriting he'd read the number back to me correctly, and he'd given me his business card, embossed with a bluebottle so lifelike I'd tried to swipe it away.

Back in my trouser suit and my tedious role as a junior executive officer in the Civil Service, I felt that our time at Annaghmakerrig was distant and unreal. I was working at a conference in Dublin Castle, but was entirely detached from where I was and what I was meant to be doing. I was longing to hear from Charlie.

Feeling reckless (and acutely bored by the conference), I pulled out my phone and sent him a text: 'We I miss you.' It didn't make sense in this context – it was the title of one of his paintings about a childhood friend who had died – but I thought he would like that I'd remembered. Then I turned off my phone so I wouldn't hear him not reply. When the first round of speakers had finished and all the delegates swarmed out for coffee break, I turned it back on. Two missed calls and three texts from Charlie. He said he'd tried to phone but kept getting a strange man's voice (he hadn't deciphered my writing after all), he asked when he could see me again, he said he missed me too.

Several weeks later my newly ex-boyfriend of seven years left the house that we had lived in together and set off to his native Newcastle-upon-Tyne in a Ford Transit van. We were both in tears. He had proposed to me six months earlier and I had said no; we had had a tumultuous time together since, and my weeks at Annaghmakerrig, even the days before I got to know Charlie, had given me the clarity of mind and the courage I needed to say goodbye. When I went back indoors, I found a note on the kitchen table beside an undrunk cup of tea. It was an invoice for 3,000 euros – he'd kept careful track of all the money he'd spent on me over the course of our relationship, and this was what he estimated I owed him.

Charlie drew lines under things too. He and his ex-wife divided furniture and books, and Charlie and Skippy moved to a small house in the village of Dalkey, south of Dublin.

Several evenings a week I would stay on the train past my stop, Sydney Parade, and travel on to Dún Laoghaire station. Charlie would cycle along Sandy-cove seafront to meet me. I would disembark grumpy and exhausted, the way long days of doing nothing can make you. At work I had begun to take a note-book and pen with me to the toilets, where I would sit in a locked cubicle and write until the energy-saving lights went off and I had to feel my way out of the room, and I would create character descriptions of my colleagues while I was meant to be taking minutes at meetings.

My role in the Civil Service was vague and unchallenging – I was a part-time, exceptionally poor proofreader and a secretary of sorts. I had got the position through a temping agency when I first moved home to Dublin after six years of an unsuccessful career as a desk editor in various publishing houses in London. The only reason I was still here five years later was that I was too insignificant to get rid of; the paltry savings that would have been made if I'd been let go wouldn't have been worth the hassle of firing me. Stuffing envelopes in your first job at nineteen is all very well, but I was still stuffing them at thirty-five. Occasionally a stranger passing by on the street outside would glance in the window and see me there, employed in this task, and I would wonder if they thought it seemed slightly odd, that there was something not quite right with me. There was nothing wrong with the Civil Service in itself – I liked all my colleagues, there was a career ladder to climb and days off for shopping at Christmas – it was just that I knew I was meant to be writing.

When I was sure it was Charlie – doing lazy circles along the promenade on his black bicycle – I would start to jog towards him. I couldn't wait to be with him and I wanted to hear all about his days. They usually involved the rescue of some sick or injured animal: an abandoned greyhound, a dying crow. Sometimes he would pull up in his car instead. More than once there was a seal he'd just saved from Killiney Beach sitting upright and curious in the passenger seat beside him, and in front of them on the dashboard, Skippy stretched out and asleep.

This tenderness towards sick and vulnerable animals came from his early life in the North. Charlie grew up in a family where not just dogs but ferrets and white mice too were tolerated. He and his big brother bred the mice in a shed in the courtyard of their home and sold them to other small boys for one shilling and sixpence – it was quite a lucrative business, Charlie said. And he took his ferret, Butch, everywhere in an old blue duffel bag, even sometimes to the cinema.

Butch liked to follow Charlie's mother around their boarding house as she served breakfast to guests. One evening he crawled into a honeymoon couple's bed and was discovered curled up asleep in their pyjamas. The outraged couple's protests fell on unsympathetic ears. 'It's only an old ferret,' Charlie's mother said. 'If you don't like it, you can leave.'

If Charlie came to meet me on foot, he would have his stick in one hand, for rhythmic strolling and for the prodding of things, and an assortment of rubbish in the other – usually beer cans and cigarette cartons that he had gathered from the shore, cursing at the laziness and ignorance of others, while he waited for me to arrive. He would walk by the sea several times a day. He said it brought him to a Zen-like state, gave him a clarity and a peace that he needed for his work; but he didn't paint pretty seascapes, he was more interested in the sea's darkness, its force and its mystery, in how people can have fun in it but how they can die in it too. He would often begin a painting with no intention of including the sea, and halfway through the tide would come in. He couldn't tolerate something so primal being made ugly and dirty with rubbish.

'Excuse me, sir!' he would shout after a stranger. 'I think you've forgotten something.' And the stranger would stop, do a quick check in their pockets for their wallet and their phone and be about to walk on when Charlie would point at the offending piece of litter with his stick and stand and watch as they returned, red-faced, to pick it up. 'Too right,' he would say to me with a little satisfied tilt of his chin as I stood in embarrassed silence beside him.

If the evening was bright, we might meet at Teddy's and share an ice-cream. Once he cajoled me onto the back of his beloved Moto Guzzi motorbike. As we roared along the coast road – him in his black helmet and shades; me in a white helmet, blonde hair flying out behind, arms gripped round his waist, wearing his too-big leather jacket and screaming – I knew that we were a cliché, that I was part of an image that he wanted to project, but I didn't mind, I was flattered that he had chosen me to complete the picture. He deliberately drove too fast, went too low around bends, shouting through the wind at me to lean with him – but I would be leaning in the opposite direction, trying frantically to keep us upright.

Charlie found my terror entertaining; he liked to scare people. When he was a boy and his parents were out at a 'do', he would lie waiting for them on the floor in the hall for several hours, tomato ketchup seeping from his head, eyes heavenward, tongue lolling out. 'Ach, don't be so stupid, Charles,' his mother would say as she stepped over him when they finally got back.

Sometimes I would make my own way to his house,

once with the ridiculously heavy gift of a watermelon, and there he would be at the door, soapy clean, eyes bright with excitement, looking suntanned and cool in a white vest, beads, loose plaid shirt, John Prine playing in the background, a double vodka in his hand. There were always small surprises at Charlie's place: blueberries in the bottom of my drink, the glass itself never regular either, sometimes embossed with a wasp or a dragonfly, or painted with flowers, his mugs decorated with Day of the Dead skulls. The table would be set for dinner and though there were only ever the two of us, we never sat side by side – Charlie would be up at one end, and I would be all the way down at the other, like a medieval king and queen. A bunny rabbit or some other stuffed toy would join us, propped up somewhere in the middle. By the fire there might be a strangely shaped piece of timber he'd found on the beach that day, or a branch or some unusual stones – never like the ones I selected, disappointingly dull without the sea's sheen by the time I got them home. He would display what he'd found in little still-life scenes around the house and garden, alongside ancient childhood toys or one of his human skulls.

Some evenings Bullet might drop round to see us.

A small, tan terrier from next door with a sharp face and pointed ears, he would shoot through the back door, skitter across the kitchen and living room, and leap on up the stairs, ricocheting against the walls and expelling little squirts of pee as he went. A quick sniff and scan and back down he would charge and up onto the sofa, where he would stay panting and still for a swift rub of his soft, warm, heaving belly; then he was down and away again like a shot, back through the house and out through the garden hedge. 'Don't move,' Charlie would sometimes say if he saw Bullet at the window, all alert and wanting to be let in, when we were on our way up to bed. And we would stand stock still for several minutes, not daring to speak, so that the dog wouldn't spot us and would think there was no one home.

There was always someone tucked into bed before I got there – Sweet Pea or Beanbag or Ted, the bear he's had since he was a baby and that goes to bed with him still. Kewpie dolls stared down at us from door frames and high shelves, huge-eyed, plump and naked. Toys watched us from his paintings too; he used them as symbols of happy times before the Troubles began, of a happy childhood by the sea.

I was once in the bathroom mid-pee when I became aware of the sound of lapping water. I looked over into the bathtub to see Skippy paddling about, stretching and flexing her rough reptilian skin. After her bath, Charlie towelled her down and swaddled her like a terrifying newborn. Then he'd put her back in her cage where she was kept warm with a heat lamp, camouflaged by foliage, with space and branches to climb on and pak choi in a bowl for her tea. At night he would make her a hot-water bottle and put it under her belly to keep her cosy. He would give her dewlap a quick scratch – 'Poor wee Skip', he'd say. Then he would cover her cage with a dark Indian throw to let her know it was time for sleep.

*

The opening bars of *Coronation Street* were the theme tune of our lives that first year, the depressing wail of the cornet an eternal comfort to us. We often talked the whole way through a half-hour episode, me curled up on the sofa, a bowl of rhubarb crumble and custard on my lap, Charlie on his knees in front of the fire, breaking sticks and moving hunks of wood about to help them dry. Charlie had watched *Corrie* with his mother as a teenager. She was always at home, always baking, always force-feeding him Battenberg cake, though he hated the stuff. He had been a large and robust baby weighing a full fourteen pounds at birth, apparently, but he said he'd been losing weight ever since. He'd even talked about changing his name to 'Slim' Whisker, he liked the sound of it. His mother used cake to try to fatten him up; there were about six meals a day in his house, three main ones and Battenberg cake in between, always presented on a paper doily.

I loved listening to Charlie's memories of his childhood; his use of language, his original turn of phrase. The words he chose were always the perfect ones for whatever he was describing, bringing images alive in my mind, his long-dead mother back to life.

'Yoo-hoo! Margery,' she would call to her friend on steep and windy Bangor High Street.

'Yoo-hoo!' Margery would call back.

'Listen, what do you think about all that palaver in the *Spectator* yesterday?'

'It's shockin', so it is, it really is shockin', the dirty brutes.'

'Dirty brutes is right. I have to go now and get a wee bit of liver from Mawhinney's, but Florrie is coming over on Tuesday for afternoon tea – why don't you come and join us?'

'I'd love to do that. I haven't seen Florrie in ages. What time?'

'Around three?'

'OK, that's lovely, I'll bring a wee sponge.'

And there were stories about Mrs French, a 'short sweet old dear who dispensed spuds, fags and marrowfats' to the locals from her little shop on the corner of Victoria Road, with its well-worn wooden counter and its glass jars of sweets. Charlie would occasionally be rewarded with a penny lump or a brandy ball along with the packet of Gallagher's Blue that his mum had sent him for. Other times, a portion of the counter would lift up like a drawbridge, and he would scurry through to see his friend Arnold. Behind this little shop, with a mouth full of penny lump, in another minuscule setting, he and Arnold would watch the continuing adventures of Robin Hood, William Tell and the Lone Ranger. Charlie was the Range Rider and Arnold was the Cisco Kid. They were going to meet in Durango when they grew up.

Sometimes Charlie was Commander-in-Chief – from the safety of the dock at Bangor Bay he would send Arnold, second-in-command, down to the pier and time him as he climbed over and under the broken wooden stays to place a 'bomb' that Charlie had fashioned out of an empty cake box from the Whistling Kettle café. Poor Arnold never made it in the time allotted and back on the dock he would be stripped of his badges and demoted.

But as Charlie grew older he lost touch with Arnold, and soon Mimi Conway was all he could think about. She was everything a pubescent boy could want, but Charlie knew she was trouble. Her boyfriend was 'a mean fucker from the back streets'. On Saturday mornings, at the Tonic Cinema Teenage Show, where they spent most of the two hours smoking and 'lumbering' girls, Charlie got the word from 'Coke' McKeown that Mimi wanted to lumber him. He remembered their big sloppy wet kisses and gum swapping, the smell of her perfume, her heat, the lacquer in her hair, the static of her cheap black jumper, a lingering BO.

My favourite of Charlie's childhood memories was the one about the Fifth Bangor Sea Scouts when they travelled to Grasmere in the Lake District, taking the boat to Heysham and then a train on to the Lakes. The court case concerning *Lady Chatterley's Lover* had ended, and the paperback had been released to the nation and was now available in bookshops, libraries, to order by post (in plain brown wrappers) and from the little kiosk on the railway platform at Heysham where the Sea Scouts were waiting for the train to Lake Windermere. Despite the steep price of three shillings and sixpence, every boy bought a copy. The bravest went first, ordering cigarettes as well and making additional book and magazine purchases for smaller boys, waiting anxiously in the distance. The Scoutmasters had been distracted by a tea-and-sandwich kiosk and were unaware of the sudden Scout interest in English literature further along the platform, or the keenly anticipated night ahead tucked up in their sleeping bags with torches, extra batteries and a good book. It was one of the 'sixers' who noticed lights glowing inside the canvas tents, where the boys were happily pleasuring themselves. Every copy of *Lady Chatterley's Lover* was confiscated. There followed a burning of the books, Charlie and the other Scouts forced to stand in salute while they watched their investment go up in flames.

*

Charlie and I were always together but alone in that first year; we didn't need anyone else. Neither of us was yet ready to introduce our friends and families to someone new. We existed in our own little bubble of bliss; I was a happy captive, pampered, soaking behind blinds in deep baths, being fed and entertained by the fire with the lights down and curtains drawn.

I began to read obituaries in *The Irish Times* – but only the very first line. All I wanted to establish was what age that person had been when they had died – if they were significantly older than Charlie I would take comfort in this and try to reassure myself, as I cried at the thought of life without him, that both of his parents had lived till they were into their late eighties. Then I would calculate the age of our yet-to-exist baby to see how long he or she would have with Charlie as their father.

I shaved Charlie's head once a week in the back garden, Skippy at our feet or up a nearby tree, always a dog somewhere. Charlie released my hair from its stubby ponytail and told me I should let it grow, he took me shopping for new, more flattering clothes. Almost daily he would produce long lists of unusual words for me to use in my writing, or a book of poetry or literature that he would read to me aloud so that I would listen and learn. He suggested laser eye surgery to correct my myopia. If I was going to be a writer I would need to see the world clearly, he said. In the days before the procedure he had winced and hopped about the sitting room gripping his nether regions at the thought of my corneas being sliced open, but he took perfect care of me during my recovery, when for twenty-four hours I felt that there was grit in my eyes and the world looked smeared with Vaseline. He was fascinated by the transformation, by the blurred becoming sharp.

I was still doing the same job, still not writing enough, but I was changing, and Charlie was encouraging this change. In some ways he was creating it. I was like one of his blank canvases, and he was making his mark.

And I felt that I was helping and changing him too. He said I gave him energy – he began getting up earlier in the mornings and painted all day while I was gone.

*

We didn't argue that first year, not even once, though we are both argumentative – Charlie admitted to occasional angry outbursts in the past, and I could sulk for several days. We were still 'in love' and had barely got to know each other yet, but there was a melancholy I saw in Charlie, even in those early days, that I began to realize stemmed specifically from one incident a long time ago. He had witnessed a murder thirty years earlier. His voice still wavered when he spoke about it and I knew that he hadn't got over it, and never fully would. The darkness and deep sadness that were evident in every one of his paintings were still inside him somewhere.

We were sitting together on the sofa one evening when Charlie told me about Michael Browne. Skippy was stretched out behind us, dreaming of whatever iguanas dream about, and Charlie had slid his cold hand between my leg and the sofa, to wedge me, as he'd say.

'Everyone understands about the Twelfth of July,' he said, looking at me sidelong with a raised and questioning eyebrow as if to continue, 'at least, they *should*.' 'But a lot goes on the night before.' I really understood so little about the North; I was born the year the Troubles began and all I recall of the early days were Gerry Adams's voice being muted on TV and being told we couldn't go out to play because of a riot at the British Embassy. Charlie told it to me a little differently that night, but he recounted it again later for a radio interview:

'The eleventh of July is a kind of tribal gathering of the clans: a lot of drinking, a lot of bravado, a lot of evil and some fun. I came across something that night that I can't forget: the murder of a sixteen-year-old boy in my home town. I came across it quite by chance and subsequently became involved in it.

'I'd been drinking in Lynch's pub in Bangor and decided to go on with some friends to a bonfire in the largely Protestant working-class estate of White-hill. It was as I was walking home that night, back towards Bangor town centre through a wooded area known as Pigeon Wood, or locally as "Pidgy", that I saw in the moonlight two young men dragging a boy into a small clearing. The men held the boy down and shot him three times in the face. Then they ran away into the dark of the trees.

'I tried to comfort him. His face was gone, the back of his head had come off in my hand. He was still alive but he wasn't conscious. I recognized him as the kid brother of a friend of mine. I remember his bony chest, the tattoos on his arm, the direction of his feet. I was in shock, I was crying, I was laughing, the whole gamut of emotions, it was like being thrown into a dishwasher, turned upside down. He was only sixteen years old. I was twenty-five. I held him while he died. It took twenty minutes. After another ten minutes the police came through the park in their Land Rovers and found us. I was covered in blood and brain.'

The police drove Charlie around the Whitehill estate the following day and Charlie identified the men he had seen – he recognized the bright yellow 'loons' (flared trousers) one of them was wearing. The two killers, David Blair and Colin Graham, were in their early twenties. They had apparently been given a firearm and orders to 'shoot a Catholic' by older elements in the local Red Hand Commando paramilitary group, which was linked closely to the UVF.

'It was the murder of an innocent as far as I was concerned,' Charlie's account went on. 'But what I saw was not unique, hundreds if not thousands of people have seen the same and worse. The tragedy is beyond the individual, the tragedy is in the family and in the friends, in the survivors. It's a great, dark, bleak period in the history of a country that I love very much, Northern Ireland, which I grew up in very happily, which was a wonderful place to be. Bangor was a thriving seaside resort and in Belfast there had been real commerce, real industry. A curtain was pulled over it in the sixties and it hasn't been pulled fully back yet.

'A hard, hard man came up to me in a pub in Bangor one night. I was eating an apple. He grabbed it from me, took a bite and spat it back out in my face. "Get the fuck out of Ireland," he said.'

Charlie had to leave Northern Ireland and his teaching job because of serious threats from the Red Hand Commando. He went to Kilburn in London and found another teaching job there. The Loyalist threats continued even there, but Charlie was undeterred and came back to Belfast to give evidence at the trial. Just before the trial, the two men changed their plea to guilty and were duly sentenced, served their time and now live in Bangor again.

'When I go back to Bangor now, I walk through the park where Michael died. I find the spot where he fell and sit down there and think of him,' Charlie concluded.

Although the details of Michael's death were horrifying, I found it hard to feel any emotion about the murder; it was totally unimaginable to me – as cold as a newspaper headline of a faraway war. And when Charlie talked about Michael, as he did quite regularly, it was Charlie's pain that upset me rather than the horror of the actual death, something so brutal yet so remote, something that I simply could not relate to.

Many years afterwards, Charlie confronted his memory of the night of the murder in a purely narrative painting depicting the killing of a teenage boy by two young men. With the family's permission he displayed it in an exhibition. This served as a form of therapy for Charlie. He worked on the details of the night it happened, got them out of his head and onto the canvas in a way that recounting the story never had. It also helped other people who were familiar with Charlie's work – it served as a sort of index, a clue to what happens in his other paintings, which don't directly deal with it but in which it often features symbolically.

Charlie had another exhibition during our early years together and that painting appeared again. It was the very same painting, on the same canvas, but in this new version he had painted the men out so that all that was left was a patch of soft green ground between trees. He called the painting *Petrichor*. I liked the word too and what it described: the smell of the air after rainfall. I would use it in my first book.

When Charlie returned the following morning to the scene where the boy had died, he found cigarette butts and matches from where he'd been smoking while he'd tried to keep him alive. Afterwards he used a burnt match in his paintings as a personal reminder of Michael, for a light gone out too quickly. This burnt matchstick is still there, sometimes prominent, sometimes tiny and hiding, in every one of his paintings.

4

Often in the evenings as Charlie set about making a fire for us, I would sit cross-legged on the floor beside him holding a piece of my writing that, after weeks of editing and reworking, I had deemed ready to show to him. I would stutter excuses and clarifications before I handed over my work, which was never anything substantial, sometimes just a few paragraphs – I wrote slowly and self-consciously at the start – but his reaction to it would dictate how the rest of the evening would go, sometimes the rest of the week.

While he read my opening sentences, I would study his face, waiting for a nod of recognition, the beginnings of a smile. Then I would get too tense and I would have to leave the room. From somewhere else in the house or the garden I would replay what I'd written in my head, word by word – having laboured over it for so long, I knew it by heart – now hating something that had seemed so clever and right an hour earlier. At weekends he would take my work with him back to bed, and I would trudge up and down the stairs with snacks and cups of tea, hoping to find him animated and engrossed by my creativity.

The role of teacher sat comfortably with Charlie. He taught fine art from 1981 to 1987 (years when I was still at school) at the National College for Art and Design (NCAD) in Dublin. Everyone said he was an excellent, though terrifying, teacher; he drove a hearse – not a station wagon, but an actual hearse – wore a long, German car coat and carried a stick with him into lessons. He was harsh with his students, unless he found them pretty or funny or cute – in which case he was even harsher, tearing up their work in front of them, making them stay back after class. I couldn't imagine ever being frightened of Charlie – this all sounded like playfulness to me; when I listened to his descriptions of his past self they seemed tongue-in-cheek rather than pretentious. I didn't understand his influences or the persona he was trying to create, but I liked that he was so different; that he had always been an eccentric, a little strange.

'Brilliant!' he would very occasionally say after

reading a couple of pages of my work, and I would see it all ahead of me: I was a talented, original writer on the cusp of incredible things. 'It's not really there, Bunt,' was his more usual response, calling me by my childhood nickname, and I would feel sick and silly and hopeless for days afterwards, sulking at him for being so blunt though I always asked him to be honest.

He gave me books to read – David Sedaris, Bill Bryson, Joan Didion – and I would study them, underlining in pencil phrases I liked, circling words I couldn't immediately use in a sentence so that I could look them up later, writing notes in the margins and putting pencil stars beside any technique or device that I thought helped to move the story along. I had never read as a child. I had lived in a house so full of books – both my parents were lifelong readers – that I took them for granted. It was a form of rebellion to refuse to engage with them. It was only when I snuck a copy of *The Thorn Birds* from my mother's bedside table at around the age of twelve that I began to develop an interest (and that was mainly because of the bits describing sex). Now, I had a lot of books to get through.

Working this way together for several months –
me writing, Charlie criticizing, me beginning again – I
produced the first three chapters. Of what, I wasn't
sure – I had no clear idea of how to continue – but I
gave it the working title of *With My Lazy Eye* and sent
it away to several Irish publishers and literary agents,
hoping that their reactions would motivate me to get
the rest of it written.

Three days later I received a phone call from
Antony Farrell at Lilliput Press, a small independent
publisher based in Dublin's Stoneybatter. He said that
he loved what he'd read and asked if he could see the
rest. He sounded a little disappointed when I told him
the rest of it didn't yet exist, but he wanted to meet me
all the same. I ran down to the kitchen to tell Charlie;
he lifted me into his arms (cursing at the heft of me),
kissed me and tried to swing me around, dropping me
early and putting a hand to his lower back in pretend
pain. We'd done it! We would celebrate that night
with double *Corrie* and a bottle of ice-cold Prosecco.

*

Charlie and I moved in together shortly after I
secured my first modest book deal, in the spring of

2006. We rented an ivy-covered Georgian house in Sandycove that was far too grand for a first-time author and an artist trying to establish himself after years abroad, but we were both impractical and we loved the idea of living and working by the sea. We turned one of the reception rooms downstairs into Charlie's studio, where he began painting large, colourful, confident pieces, Lucinda Williams crooning away while he worked. I took six weeks' unpaid leave from the Civil Service and wrote full time from the bedroom above him – coming downstairs to have him read things, meeting him in the kitchen for coffee and to eat lunch. In the late afternoons, when we'd both had enough, we would go through a yellow wooden gate at the end of the garden, framed for most of the year with white clematis, and down a grassy laneway that led to the rocks and the sea. We liked it best by Bulloch Harbour, watching fishermen feed gulls in a grey and screaming frenzy, dogs rolling in fish juice, brightly coloured overturned wooden boats along the oily slipway.

Charlie knew about the sea; this was his domain. He knew the names of all the seabirds, he could spot a seal's slick head in the water before anyone else, he knew the best vantage points from which to take a photograph, he chatted easily to anyone we met. And then home again to make a fire and drink and talk and watch TV and early to bed, where Charlie slept so utterly still and straight I would have the feeling that he was awake, though he would tell me, the next morning, about the wild dream he'd had of killing Gerry Adams. Then he would laugh and pull me towards him and say that he'd missed me while he was sleeping.

With Charlie's edits, Antony's guidance, the panicky pressure of someone believing in me, and the knowledge that I could so easily fuck it all up, I worked harder than I had on anything before and the novel began to take shape.

It was Charlie's idea to include photographs, taking inspiration from the works of W. G. Sebald. We chose them together and he dropped the uncaptioned images into the text and spread them irregularly throughout the book: childhood photos, pictures of broken glasses, doves, dragonflies. He took a break from painting and worked for weeks on these – though he found them fiddly and irritating – while I sat upstairs, writing.

Julia Kelly

Time passed, I completed a first draft and I was sitting once again on my swivel seat in my Civil Service office, when an email from Antony slithered into my inbox. Several weeks earlier he had sent galleys out to some authors, including my favourite writer, John Banville, requesting an endorsement.

'Will this do?' John Banville had replied, followed by his quote:

Julia Kelly's is surely the freshest voice in Irish fiction since the wonderful early novels of Edna O'Brien. This is a future to watch.

Hot-faced and shaking, I phoned my mother. I read the quote out to her at least three times, varying my emphasis for impact. What I heard in her voice, beyond pride, beyond joy, was pure and overwhelming relief. I'd been a needy and confused child who wanted to be a boy until the age of fourteen, when I suddenly wanted to be *with* boys. I was a pain in the backside throughout my teenage years – one school report was so appalling that it made my father roll the 'r' in rotten (a strange and alarming sound and a signal that I needed to make a run for it). To a man who spoke five languages and was so brilliant during his own schooldays that he was known as 'the professor',

I was an endless source of frustration.

'I wouldn't mind if you were stupid,' he'd roar as he walked away from me and back down the stairs into his study while I sat cross-legged in front of my bedroom mirror applying kohl liner to my lids, fighting tears. When I failed my first year at college, he said it would take all his influence to get me a job at the checkout in Tesco. He later modified this to packing bags at the same supermarket; I agreed – my grasp of maths wasn't strong enough for the till. Since then, I had been gently encouraged to leave or openly fired from every job I'd had. My mother had been wearily defending me for years, over the slam of my father's fist on the kitchen table. After he died, she continued to support and encourage every new venture or idea I had. Perhaps now, at last, her strange and awkward daughter would achieve something in her life.

It took Xanax washed down with a double vodka – Charlie introduced me to both of these things – to get me through my first reading. The transition from solitary months of writing quietly at home to having to be media savvy and bright and shiny and self-promoting wasn't one I made easily. I didn't feel confident of what I had to say, or that I had much to say at all. I worried that I had no imagination: I wrote from my own life, found plots impossible and had grown to hate narrative arcs. I was still on the steepest learning curve, I still felt like a fraud.

I froze in front of six hundred people at Dún Laoghaire Town Hall, where the author Joseph O'Connor and I were each reading from our new books. The reading itself had gone smoothly enough; I had rehearsed endlessly in front of Charlie and was in a medicated calm. Charlie was there – he was always there, rooting for me, sitting back, arms folded, one leg crossed over the other, the way thin men sit. He was not just my partner: he was my mentor, my second agent, a director assessing my performance, taking mental notes for a debrief when we got home.

The evening was almost over. We were at the question-and-answer part, which I hated.

'Was there any particular book that inspired you as a teenager?' a woman in the front row asked, lips pursed expectantly, waiting to be entertained by my response.

I couldn't think of a single book. There was *The Thorn Birds* of course, but I felt I couldn't say that. It wasn't literary enough; it would just seem weird, not right. So I said nothing at all, not a word. I simply passed the microphone to Joe sitting beside me.

'For me it was definitely *The Catcher in the Rye*.'

'Oh, oh!' I said, snatching it back from him. 'That was my one too! *The Catcher in the Rye*, that's just what I was going to say. It had a very profound influence on me.' Even as I spoke I was telling myself to remember Charlie's advice: 'Take a thought once round your head before expressing it.' I sought him out in the audience, knowing already that he wouldn't meet my eye – I was just too painful to watch, to listen to, too excruciating. Sure enough, he had his head deep in his hands and I dreaded the conversation we would have on the journey home. It would begin with laughter, as it always did, but through his teasing, he would make his disappointment clear and I would go to bed tearful and embarrassed.

Having my photograph taken was a further ordeal. I wanted to appear earnest, pensive – Joan Didion in a black polo neck, New York in the seventies. I turned out more like Miss Piggy: big lipsticky smile, bouncy hair, a dress showing too much cleavage. Photographers were always disappointed when they arrived at the house to find me in a sweatshirt and jeans. They would encourage me to change into something more glamorous and to smile at the camera rather than gaze, preoccupied, into the distance – my preference, as it disguised my lazy eye and made me look a little more serious. Charlie watched and stage-managed, adding interesting objects in the background: a stag's antlers, a heavy iron cross, a human skull. The result was inevitably bizarre.

With My Lazy Eye won Newcomer of the Year at the Irish Book Awards that year, and I got a call one Friday evening from Antony to say that a UK publishing house, Quercus, had bought my book from Lilliput and had offered me a two-book deal.

*

There was never any jealousy from Charlie. I was his protégée, and he stood proud beside me – boasting about my achievements, abandoning his studio and taking long walks with me on days when interviews didn't go well. He saw my book's success as a reflection on himself – he had guided and directed me throughout. I needed to have him beside me; I felt that he was the interesting one – the one with the good stories, the one who was rewarding company at literary lunches and author events. Even though sometimes I was huffy and rebellious towards Charlie, I invariably came round to his way of thinking. I still wanted to learn from him, and he still wanted to teach and improve me. We lived very harmoniously like this.

It helped that Charlie's own work was doing so well. He had a sell-out one-man show at the Solomon Gallery in Dublin that autumn. Van Morrison bought the first painting, before the show had officially opened, and by the time Bono got there he said all the ones he wanted had already been sold.

Charlie loved music and musicians. He didn't have a lot of empathy for other visual artists, and he didn't like to sit around talking about art, but he loved to talk about music. He had a huge music collection and an incredibly broad knowledge of country, jazz and blues. When I first met Charlie I thought he was trying to impress me when he mentioned his famous friends – and in part he probably was – but to him they really were just people he happened to have met in the course of his life and work. He had travelled through America with Van Morrison and still met him for the occasional 'Ruby Murray' (that's a curry) or a coffee locally. And Charlie had first met the members of U2 when he worked with Windmill Lane recording studios in Dublin in the early nineties, where he made music videos. In the mid-nineties, he and another director, Meiert Avis, went out to California and set up Windmill Lane in Santa Monica. The studios were in a cavernous factory a few blocks from Santa Monica's downtown. Enormous B-52 bomber wing flaps divided the office space, where ejector seats served as chairs and paintings and sculpture, along with three of Meiert's electric guitars, adorned the exposed brick walls.

Charlie moved to LA then with his wife, Mariad, and their two young daughters, India and Domino, and spent nine years working as a computer painter, producing painterly effects as an overlay or canvas for rock videos. He was known as Windmill's 'artist in residence' because of the irregular hours he worked – he liked to arrive late after a walk on the beach in the mornings and to knock off for the day around three o'clock so he could go home for a swim. He focused exclusively on the projects that interested him and struggled with some of the technology. This and his light work schedule caused resentment among his work colleagues, but he was having a wonderful life in the sunshine, living on the beach at Pacific Palisades, enjoying the San Bernardino mountains and the desert.

I loved to listen to Charlie talk about his life in California. He missed it daily – the nature, the heat, the light. We pored over photo albums: Charlie beside his vintage Chevrolet Impala, with a deep suntan and wearing a Stetson, with dogs, rabbits, reptiles around him. Even repeating aloud the names of the places he'd lived in and seen gave him pleasure, and I loved the sound of the words: Big Sur, San Luis Obispo, Pasadena, Carmel.

Charlie loved to go back to places he'd been to before, and he loved when I travelled with him so he could show me around and ply me with stories and information. In February 2008 when he was asked to exhibit at a pre-Oscars event, he took me to California with him. He worked for months to put a show together and paid vast amounts to have twenty paintings shipped from Dublin to a theatre in Los Angeles, where we spent two full days together hanging them.

The evening, which began in a crazy flash of cameras and people calling Charlie's name, didn't go as we'd hoped: no one was interested in looking at art and certainly not in purchasing it – they all wanted to network, to make connections, to sell themselves – and he sold almost nothing on the night. I knew that he was terribly disappointed and embarrassed, but his reaction was to laugh about it dismissively and to carry on with our holiday. He took me to his old house on The Bluffs in Pacific Palisades, from where he had spent happy days watching Pamela Anderson being filmed for *Baywatch* on the beach below. We drove along the Pacific Coast Highway, stopping to watch blubbery elephant seals fighting on the beach, and through the bohemian enclave of Topanga Canyon: streams, waterfalls, cliffs of exposed bedrock, chaparral-covered hills. We toured Hearst Castle overlooking the village of San Simeon and had a drink at the beautifully pink and tacky Madonna Inn in San Luis Obispo.

Then we went east into the arid uplands: we lay out on huge flat boulders at Joshua Tree where the Mojave and Lower Colorado deserts join to form a national park, we visited Point Dume on the coast of Malibu at the far end of Santa Monica Bay, where we saw a school of grey whales. It was on this day, with Charlie walking ahead, full of chat and stories and facts, in the torpid heat of the late afternoon, feeling the sun warm on the back of my neck, the pleasant tickle of long grass about my ankles, cicadas making a racket in the cottonwood trees, that I felt a moment of pure happiness. It was fleeting, the way happiness is – even as I acknowledged it, it became diluted by other things like worry that it would not last – but it was there at that moment. I was truly happy.

I watched everything on that holiday, took notes, listened to Charlie's language, his gift for describing things, the vivid pictures he painted, his words and language always, in my eyes, so perfectly selected and right.

*

Charlie's friends, made up largely of musicians and artists, seemed a little wary of me at the start. I know how I looked to them – much younger than Charlie (and than his ex-wife), blonde, with a Dublin 4 address and therefore, indisputably, privileged and unlikely to be kind or decent or creative and very unlikely to have had any suffering in my life. With some of them I felt boxed and labelled before I'd had a chance to speak. His friends were a tight and insular group and there was a twitchy and protective ring around the king and the queen, Bono and Ali Hewson. Charlie had been given the nickname of 'Happy' Whisker, because he was often so glum, but they were very fond of him and supportive, and were impressed by his talents and his musical knowledge.

There were many, many art openings, in those first few years I spent with Charlie, and parties and dinners and night swimming on the beach on New Year's Eve or in the heated pool at the Hewsons' house on Christmas Day. We tied wishes to Chinese lanterns and watched them float up over Killiney Bay. There were games of tennis on the courts in the garden, dizzy with champagne, once to an audience of Javier Bardem and Penelope Cruz in which, with a lot of cursing and a professional grunt, I served four games of double faults. I'd played a lot as a teenager and refused to serve underarm, though I was mortified and my partner was unimpressed at the result. I was a terrible combination of very competitive and not very good, especially when I knew I was being watched.

When U2 played in New York in the autumn of 2005, Charlie and I flew over to go to some of their shows. It was a blurry, alcohol-drenched week of torrential rain. They sent stretch limousines to collect us from our hotel and deliver us dry to Madison Square Garden, where we were hurried through the backstage area and out into the cool air of the huge stadium – the euphoric, pulsating groove of Arcade Fire and the building buzz of the audience around us – to the mixing desk, our Access All Areas badges dangling from our chests, both of us adopting a slightly nonchalant air, not wanting our excitement to show.

One night that week we were taken to Babbo's restaurant in Greenwich Village for an after-show party where we shared a table with Scarlett Johansson, Jay Z, Moby, Woody Harrelson, Helena Christensen and Christy Turlington. Bono was sitting beside me, as silly, fun and warm as ever, doing an excellent impression of George W. Bush. We got giddy, Charlie kissed Scarlett Johansson on the lips, I called Moby a dick (unintentionally). Bono asked if he could see some of my writing, and we spoke about Charlie and me – I remember telling him I would top myself if anything ever happened to Charlie; it may have sounded like drunken exaggeration, but at that moment I meant it honestly, unreservedly. I simply could not imagine the bleakness of life without Charlie.

Bono was endlessly encouraging of Charlie, that night introducing him to the owner of the most prestigious gallery in New York as 'one of Ireland's finest artists'. He was a collector of Charlie's works and had commissioned him, many years earlier, to design the etching on the metal gates of his Killiney home. Charlie was also fiercely loyal about Bono and his family and would defend him passionately when others put him down – which the Irish, especially and oddly, like to do.

On our way back to our hotel in the early hours the following morning, ears still ringing from the concert, voices hoarse from singing along to 'Beautiful Day', Charlie put his arm around my shoulder, pulled me closer, kissed me on the forehead and said: 'I didn't want to say anything earlier but your breath was a tiny bit sour all evening.' I sulked for a while, then I got cross – why the hell couldn't he have mentioned it a little earlier instead of watching me move in close and breathe my foul breath over everyone? We had our first fight outside Fitzpatrick's Hotel on Lexington Avenue that night in the driving rain.

*

When Charlie first met my friends and family he was his very best self. I didn't know then that there was another side to him – this was the only version of Charlie I'd ever seen. Friends said he was their favourite of all my boyfriends, one even developed a brief crush on him. When I told my big brother about Charlie and me, he invited us to dinner and Charlie took centre stage, telling childhood stories at my insistence as I sat back and listened, proud and adoring, watching my brother's and his wife's reactions to see if they saw what I saw in him. The evening ended with my brother taking out his guitar and Charlie singing Woody Guthrie's 'This Land is Your Land', the rest of us joining in for the bits we could remember. My sister-in-law sent a text the following day: 'We love Charlie,' she said. 'You could put him on Mars, and he would get along with everyone.'

This didn't turn out to be true. While Charlie remained kind and friendly to strangers – eccentric, elderly women were his favourite, and he seemed to have a radar for any human or animal in need of help – he began, not long after meeting my friends and family, to distance himself from them.

One evening we sat at our kitchen table, at the start of a bank holiday weekend with no plans. That never bothered Charlie – he was rarely aware of what day of the week it was, never partook in traditional celebrations – but I was a planner and a lover of tradition, and it felt lonely to be at a loose end. I told him that we'd been invited on a barge trip down the Shannon with two other couples, old friends of mine. I was full of adrenaline, like a child asking a parent for a big favour, knowing the answer would almost certainly be no. 'Just hear me out,' I kept having to say. So he sat silent, staring at me and when I'd finished he said: 'That sounds like absolute hell.' I pleaded with him, insisted it would be romantic and an adventure. 'Bunkum!' he said. He was nearly sixty, he had enough friends, he didn't need any more. This was our second row, more serious than the first. I told him, in tears, that I wanted him to get to know *my* friends, as I had done his, I wanted to spend time with them and I also, childishly and jealously, didn't want my friends to have fun together without me.

He would not be swayed about the barge journey, but we reached a compromise that Charlie would attend occasions that were truly important to me. On other occasions I would just have to go on my own. I began to choose carefully – I didn't want to nag or plead with him – but his list of non-negotiables grew. He refused to go to baptisms, communions or confirmations – he was an atheist and didn't agree with putting children through these ceremonies. He couldn't tolerate two seconds at a kid's party. Barbecues were out of the question – the wretched stench of burning meat made him want to 'boke' – and long slow dinners were torture, he said they made his toes curl.

When I could cajole him along to some event – Christmas Day with my family, for example, or a close friend's wedding – he would quickly get restless, and I would try to encourage him into conversation, but there would invariably be a problem. Often he would panic when some unlucky person was doing their best to engage him. He would complain to me that they were talking 'at him' or too loudly or too much and he would then be unable to eat, food would become lodged in his throat and he would have to go outside to regurgitate. I would leave my dinner and stand outside with him, rubbing his back, promising that we would go home soon. On other occasions he would get up and walk out of a restaurant quite openly and pointedly because someone had ordered *foie gras* or baby squid.

He didn't understand why I had to see my family so often – why there had to be so many goddamn celebrations, and why I had to waste my money buying birthday presents and Christmas presents for godchildren, nieces and nephews. His ex-wife had come from a large and close Catholic family too and now he was having to go through it all again. Soon funerals were all he tolerated – he always enjoyed a good funeral – but at this point in our lives these were seldom and few.

Because he wouldn't come with me and was so often miserable when he did, I began to go out alone, to parties, to dinners, to any events involving children or any religious ceremonies, but I was anxious and clock-watching from the moment I arrived. I needed to get home as soon as I could; I knew Charlie was lonely without me and if I was late he would sulk and be irritable or sometimes not talk to me at all – he would lie very still in the dark while I undressed, pretending to be asleep. I still loved him and didn't want to upset him – I wanted to curl up beside him and tell him all about my evening. His mood would thaw the following day, as soon as I had given him some attention, and we would walk together, and I would recount the details of what he'd missed.

If I mentioned any irritation I had with a friend, any small transgression, that was it – Charlie took against them for ever. They became another person on his blacklist, another reason not to go out. He was very protective towards me, but he didn't understand that I could complain about someone and yet still want to see them, still want them in my life. He told me daily that he adored me, that I was the most beautiful girl he'd ever met, and that if I left him he would walk straight into the sea.

*

As a child I had never dreamed of being married, but I was sure I wanted a baby, ideally several of them. 'Why don't you apply for a job in a crèche?' my mother would say, running out of possible career options. 'You're wonderful with children.' And I did love their company, I could do a Donald Duck impression that made them laugh, and I still often felt like a seven-year-old myself. I was in fact thirty-eight and running short of time. I began idly to talk about baby names on our daily walks – Charlie liked Arlo (after Arlo Guthrie) and Isis, inspired by Dylan's mystical child. He loved Dixie. I liked Ruben, Samuel, Saul, all the Old Testament names: not for a child of his, he said.

He told me that he had once been so dead-set against children that he described himself as being a member of the King Herod Society; but when his eldest daughter, India, was born his heart melted, and when he and Mariad had their second daughter, Domino, he began to experience joy through them. He started a collection of Sylvanian toys, made videos of his small girls talking and playing together, cycled through Dublin with one or other of them on the back of his bike.

And so, not long after we moved in together, we began to try – if this was what I really wanted, Charlie would go along with it. I believed that a baby would make things better between us, would make us a proper family and that I would be happier and more fulfilled. Leading independent social lives was a compromise I could accept, as Charlie and I were very content together, our home life was harmonious. A baby would give us something new to talk about, it would bring us closer to each other, make our commitment more solid.

After a few months of enjoyable and energetic effort, I was still not pregnant and I felt I was doing something wrong. I bought books on fertility and began to take my temperature when I woke, Charlie in bed beside me thinking that my anxiety was insane. I teased him about his swimmers being lazy – we laughed as we imagined them with snorkels, floating on their backs, taking it easy. I ate pineapples, took cough medicine, lit candles at the local church. Charlie began to get bored of it all and started to resent scheduled sex. 'Maybe you just can't have kids,' he said one evening. I lay in the dark, stunned and sobbing, but I was determined: I would do whatever it took to have a baby. I continued to try to boost my fertility. I took up yoga, had acupuncture, drank revolting herbal concoctions and tried homeopathic remedies.

Towards the end of that year, we took out a huge mortgage – wildly exaggerating our joint incomes – and bought a large red-brick Victorian home in Bray, County Wicklow. It was just the two of us now. Poor Skippy had been put down after a fall from a perch in which she fractured her back. Charlie cried aloud when he lost her; he was so distraught that for several days I could do nothing at all to comfort him. It frightened me to see him so vulnerable and low. Soon after Skippy's death and with his birthday approaching, I found and purchased a small, second-hand wooden boat – since our time on the lake at Annaghmakerrig he had talked of how much he would like to own a skiff of some kind. I employed a family friend to paint and repair it, and I met him at Bulloch Harbour one sodden Sunday morning. Together we pulled the boat on a trailer up the hill and through the yellow back gate of our home in Sandycove. And there it was, when Charlie looked out the kitchen window while waiting for the kettle to boil – a little white boat, the name *Skippy* painted in blue on its starboard side.

Charlie said the baby would come once we had our new home. This is what swans do, he said. They build their nests, line them with their own down and grasses and anything soft, so the eggs don't get damaged or crushed. They get everything ready and then they have their babies. We had four bedrooms, a long back garden with a small gated area and wooden playhouse at the end. This is where we put *Skippy* the boat. Charlie didn't feel that she was seaworthy – but it would be fun for children to play in, he said. It was a house that needed children, and the longer we lived there without them, the emptier it and I felt.

I saw the doctor, who said I talked too fast, that I needed to slow down. I went online and tried all the things that had worked for other women. I followed each of them to the letter. They didn't work. We got a dog from a rescue shelter. He'd been abandoned twice already in his short life and was so desperate for us to take him home that on the day we visited it took twenty minutes to get him calm enough to attach a lead to his collar. The shelter had called him Scamp; we renamed him Mr Blue.

And then, after almost two years of trying, of repeatedly holding a little white stick to the light with shaking hands and turning it and squinting at it, I saw the faintest of faint pink lines. I checked it and checked it again. I threw it in the bin, retrieved it ten minutes later to study and study it further. Was it? There it was! A beautiful, perfect pink line.

*

Charlie was nervous of our baby's arrival. He had felt that he was past that part of his life, and he had been looking forward to a book by the fire in the evening, a pipe, maybe, but I could not wait to meet him or her.

'I'm sure this is it, pet,' my mother said, rubbing her hands together in anticipation as she sat at the end of my bed. It was February 2009, Pancake Tuesday, and my baby was ten days late. In the morning I'd been complaining of mild cramps as I ate my jelly and ice-cream and watched *The Jeremy Kyle Show*. Perhaps I had a high pain threshold, maybe this labour thing was really no big deal.

Five hours later I was writhing in agony, on my hands and knees on the floor, my head under a chair, fluids oozing from every orifice, howling that I couldn't do it, that I'd changed my mind, that I didn't want a baby after all.

And then at 2.18 in the afternoon – such a mundane time of day – a little animated alien appeared blinking between my legs. They had to suck her out, my poor baby, she was more distressed than her mother and not the right colour, but a magician in a multicoloured waistcoat appeared, tossed her about the place and made her turn pink. She was blemish-free and perfect when he handed her to me, she even had a side part-ing and her own rhythm: nibble, nibble, nibble, as she took tiny tugs at my breast, brand-new fingers coiling and uncoiling around my thumb, new eyes trying to focus on my face.

For the first time since we met, I turned away from Charlie – my attention shifted to our child. I had found someone new to be in love with, and they needed me back. I'd put Charlie on a pedestal – he said himself that I'd been spellbound by him – and now that pedestal was abruptly removed. I was absorbed and fascinated by this brand-new human being. I was also physically drained by her. She was like an adorable little leech. After hours of breastfeeding each day and night, I had no more left to give; a milky muslin cloth where my cleavage used to be. Bed was for sleep only, and sleep became a critical, vital need. Charlie and I moved into separate rooms.

When I complained of feeling exhausted, over-whelmed, Charlie would say I was running about too much and would encourage me to cancel whatever plans I had made to meet friends and their babies for coffee or to go to baby classes or out for baby-free evenings. I told him that these people made me happy, that far from exhausting me, they gave me energy, but he couldn't see that, he felt they were just taking from me – why did I always have to travel to meet them? Why couldn't they call around to our house, he asked again and again. Because he didn't want them in our home, I told him, because they didn't feel welcome there.

When the baby was six months old, I passed my driving test – it was third time round and the licence was for an automatic car only, but now I was no longer dependent on Charlie to deliver or collect me from places, or on public transport. It gave me a feeling of independence and freedom that I didn't know I'd been lacking.

Sometimes in the mornings we would all lie together, our daughter between us, deliciously squishy and soft, tiny hands gripping tiny toes. And we would be happy, until she would start to 'nerp' – the word Charlie used for her whining. She'd whimper and roll onto her side and reach out her arms for me. Then Charlie would get up and move away or out of the room. 'She just doesn't like me,' he'd say.

Together they competed for my attention, and the baby always won. Charlie helped a lot at the start – he changed nappies, read to her from his ancient Rupert Bear annuals, shared his toy collection with her, sang to her. He gave her a dozen nicknames: Narky Nora when she grumbled, Granny McGurk when she gurned, Wee Stinky if her nappy needed changing, but most of the time Nipey or the Nipe. He carried her around the garden in his arms, holding her up to show her the detail of a spider's web, the incredible colour of a particular plant.

We tried to get back to our old pattern of work. I was always best in the mornings, Charlie preferred the afternoons, still playing his music loud; more innocent and childlike images like ladybirds began to appear on his canvases. While I wrote in the study downstairs, Charlie would hang out with the Nipe in the sitting-room above, but at the slightest whimper I would be up, not letting him get to know her, not allowing him to make mistakes. I was distrustful and critical of his abilities and this made him feel redundant, to begin to doubt himself.

When the Nipe was a year old, I began in a haphazard and half-interested way to write my second novel, about a schoolteacher travelling to California. I had visited there only briefly, twice, so I plundered Charlie's memory to try to create a believable world. I wrote in the mornings and read my work aloud to him at night. In this way I cobbled together a novel that was too short and didn't work.

I sent it off, exhausted and panicking; it was already several months late. I was disappointed, though not surprised, when it was rejected. I was missing from it, my publisher said, my voice wasn't there.

'Do you have any other ideas?' my agent asked during a tearful conversation. I was at the sitting room window, gazing out at the playground across the road, feeling desolate and uninspired. Needing an answer, I said without any forethought that I could probably write about the playground, about a mother and a child on their own. Our fictional world could centre around this place where the Nipe and I spent our afternoons. And it did feel like we were largely on our own. Charlie wanted to join in – he felt increasingly isolated – and occasionally he would try, but it was always a tense and uneasy mix. He didn't have the energy or the stamina to keep up with a very young child and instead of slowing down and walking with him, I always ran ahead to be with her.

'Look, there's Dada!' I would sometimes say, when I noticed Charlie watching us from high up in his studio opposite the playground. I'd lift Nipey out of the bucket swing and carry her closer to the park railings, and we would smile and shout over at him, me holding her small wrist to show her how to wave. Mostly he smiled and waved the paintbrush in his hand back at us. But there were days when he would stand there expressionless or move abstractedly away from the window, seeming not to have seen us at all.

5

I know that my mother is asleep. I can hear her whistling snores through the wall that separates our adjoining rooms. She may deny it in the morning – she has never liked to admit to sleep, as though it were a weakness, a taking of her eye off things, but it comes easily to her, even in her armchair as she watches television. Her snores are not rhythmic or regular – each one varies from the last in its volume and duration and there are moments of apnoea and fitful coughs in between. They compete with the drone of the air con to keep me awake.

We are staying at a hotel near Montclair, New Jersey – Charlie, Mum, two-year-old Nipey and me. It is July 2011, and we're here for a solo show of Charlie's latest work. Mum joined us on the trip, ostensibly to help mind her grandchild but really because she loves being on holiday and loves to be part of things. While she is here she makes plans for her next trip, after Christmas – to the Galapagos Islands, to see the giant tortoises. At breakfast she will talk of lunch: that's how she lives, never in the moment or in the past, always looking ahead.

I'm on a sofa bed in the sitting room. The Nipe is in the bedroom next door with her dad. After four nights of watching *Barney* in the small hours with a zingy awake toddler, my need for sleep is acute. As Charlie has always been a better sleeper than I, we all agreed that tonight he would let her share with him. I don't know the time, but it's bright enough to manoeuvre my way to the window without turning on lights. I lift the net curtain to try and gauge the hour: it still looks balmy outside, the palm trees around the floodlit pool are motionless, there are no ripples on the water. Yesterday it was a temper-fraying 110 degrees Fahrenheit, too hot to be outdoors. We'd gone instead by taxi into central Manhattan to the Guggenheim Museum.

Rather than share a lift full of sweating tourists there, we'd chosen to walk up the long spiralling ramp to the top. The Nipe, who would ordinarily complain about such a climb and stretch her arms out to be carried, was too absorbed in a private game to notice. She was bouncing her doll, 'Cloth Dolly' – a strange little toy with tufty red hair, a cloth body and hard plastic shoes – along the edge of the shallow boundary wall as we looked at art. Mum was in high good form, as she would say of herself. She had studied history of art as a mature student so she knew a thing or two, and now she was in a gallery with a real contemporary artist whom she questioned and hoped to impress, finishing his sentences in that muttery way she had, as if to say she was just about to say the same thing. Charlie was competitive about his work and dismissive of a lot of what appealed to my mum, but he wanted to show off his knowledge, and for once his child, who didn't like to be excluded, wasn't interrupting their conversation. He was always drawn to Nipey when she was quiet, her attention absorbed in something else. He snuck up behind her now, as Mum considered a piece entitled *All the Clothes of a Woman*, grabbed her round the waist and lifted her into his arms.

'Poor wee Nipey, wet and weary, sold her bed, slept in the hay. What a silly wee billy she was.' He squeezed her and gave her lots of quick little kisses on the neck. She humoured him for a moment then gave me a pleading sort of look.

'Dada! I'm dus busy doing something,' she said, struggling to be free so that she could get back to her game. Always a little hurt by her rejections, Charlie was silent for a while, but became more animated when he saw the sunlight flooding through the glass dome above us as we reached the top floor: 'Wow, look at that Tintoretto sky!' Mum and I craned our necks to see it for ourselves – and at that moment, out of bravery or boldness or both, the Nipe dangled her doll over the wall and let her go. Down she fell, all the way to the ground floor where she hit a Japanese woman on the head. When we peered over to look, the Nipe on tiptoes and crying, a dozen faces stared back up at us.

Cloth Dolly was on the floor in the centre of a gathering crowd, limbs askew, like a tiny murder victim. A security guard picked her up, sought us out in the crowd and beckoned us down. We apologized to the Japanese woman, who was being comforted by her family, Cloth Dolly was confiscated, and we were led to a room where we were interrogated for over half an hour before the doll was returned and we were encouraged out of the building. It would be funny in the future, a funny little story to tell friends, but none of us found it funny that day. We were all too hot, too irritable, too jet-lagged – and there was something wrong with Charlie.

At breakfast he had stood with an empty glass in front of the drinks dispenser, not knowing what he needed to do to get some orange juice. I watched him accept a stranger's help when they saw him standing there. And this evening he had complained again to the stiff-faced, immaculate woman at reception that the lifts weren't working, though behind us everyone else was happily ascending and descending. He got lost on his way back to our room when he went to get some water from the bar and had flung a shoe at the window in anger. He'd been asking me to order for him in restaurants all week, he couldn't understand the currency and the phone was an endless source of frustration – when he tried to dial nine for an outside line, he kept getting emergency services.

The sound of something being knocked over in the bedroom, the glug of water spilt. 'Cunt!'

I get up, turn the knob of the door. I can see our child in the slice of light I've created. She is lying across the bed in her vest and pull up, the covers kicked off as always and her little legs bent at the knee as is her habit, as though she's mid sit-up. Her eyes are closed but her mouth is working furiously at her sucky blanket. She is trying her best to stay asleep.

Charlie is standing by the wall with his hands against it, inching along as though feeling for a secret opening. He looks at me in a daze, my presence adding to his disorientation.

'Charlie, what are you doing? It's the middle of the night.'

'Ach, sweetie, there you are. I was just looking for you,' he says, with no attempt at a whisper, lunging forward to embrace me. He stubs his foot on the bed-side table.

'Fuck!'

'Be quiet,' I hiss. Not only is he about to wake our finally time-adjusted child, he is cursing in front of her.

'Where the hell is the toilet? I need a pee.' I take hold of his arm and tug him into the bathroom. I turn on the light. He farts, apologizes. I groan.

'Don't flush, OK? It'll wake her.' I leave him, creep out of the room and settle back onto the sofa bed; the springs squeak in complaint.

I turn my pillow, rest my head on its cool side and listen to Mum's snores, the air conditioning and now some new sounds: the ping of the lift, the rattle of a trolley along the corridor. Should I move Nipe back in here with me? Her dad seems drunk but he couldn't be – he had driven all of us out to dinner so hadn't been drinking the night before. I take the lazy decision.

I am resentful of our friends, a couple from Dublin, who are on the same floor as us but at the opposite end. They had travelled over to join us for the week, leaving their young daughter at home with her grand-parents, and are having a wonderful holiday of late nights and lie-ins. She told me yesterday that they'd never had such good and satisfying sex. Tomorrow they would be flown by private jet to visit rock-star friends in the Hamptons. Yesterday morning she was in bed with a hangover, and he was running about the place getting things to help make it endurable for her, while I tried to teach Charlie how to use the room key.

'He's become quite dependent on you, pet, hasn't he?' Mum had said to me the day before. This was mys-tifying to a woman who, widowed at the age of fifty, was used to doing everything for herself. She was the most practical, unflappable person I had ever known; for every problem she found a solution, in a cloudy sky she always saw the patch of blue. But Charlie's never been practical, I told her and kept telling myself, that's not what I signed up for. He's an artist, he's creative, he thinks differently. I could explain away his recent disorientation, his dependency, his inability to use money, his wild outbursts: he was drunk, he was stressed, he was older (sixty-two to my forty-two now) he was bad with jet lag, the heat was getting to him, he had always been hot-tempered, had always been dark.

At his opening he had been poised and dapper in his loose black suit and trilby hat, and so articulate as he was filmed for a local television channel; he had the interviewer laughing and nodding in recognition from the offset. He posed for photos, answered questions from enthusiastic buyers, even signed some autographs. Mum had been the first to buy a painting – one of Charlie's hens. 'Dora', I think he had named her, who would go nicely alongside 'Arnold', the hen she had purchased at his last show. The evening had gone well, lots of red stickers and several half ones, which meant that they were thinking about it. There was nothing wrong with Charlie.

'Dada? Mum!'

I get up, go back into the bedroom, turn on the light. Nipey is sitting up in bed, holding her forearm against her eyes to shield them from the stark brightness, her face crumpled with confusion. 'It's not my fault,' Charlie says, without turning around. He is standing at the side of the bed, with his boxers around his ankles. He is peeing onto the white sheets. 'I couldn't find the toilet.'

*

It's a grey afternoon in February 2012. We are at home in Dublin, eight months after our trip to the States, now a hot summer memory. A friend and her children are here to play. Charlie has been up in his studio working/hiding since they arrived – he doesn't like children who aren't his own, dismissing them universally as too noisy, too snotty, too messy. This morning he went from room to room to remove or put out of reach all of his collection of toys so that they wouldn't be touched or disturbed.

I am at the sink filling the kettle when I hear Charlie call me. I open the kitchen door, stand by the banisters and shout back at him. 'Julia?' he says again. His voice is quiet and near. I walk through the hall, stop at the bottom of the stairs. Charlie is standing at the top of them.

'Can you come up here please?'

'What's wrong? You sound strange.'

We'd just come in from the garden – my friend and I had been down at the wooden playhouse, trying to keep warm and make conversation while shunting our kids up the ladder or holding them round their waists as they hung off the monkey bars. We'd trampled back indoors when it began to get dark, mucky and cold with dog dirt on our shoes. The orangey light coming from the kitchen had cheered me. I've always disliked afternoons, am always happier in the evenings. And I'd felt disconcerted that day. My mother had set off for her trip to the Galapagos Islands a few days earlier. She wasn't fit enough, I thought, for such a long journey. I never liked her to be away and always worried about her, had a general sense of unease, until she was home again.

Has one of the kids damaged something of Charlie's? This is what I am thinking as I climb the stairs. He takes my hand and leads me in silence to the sitting room. What is he about to show me? I imagine spilled paint, broken toys, smashed vases. Nothing. Everything is normal, everything is in its place. He tells me to sit down. I sit, he sits on the coffee table opposite me, our knees are touching. I want him to do something silly, the sort of thing he does to make Nipey laugh – I want him to stand on the coffee table and balance on one leg without wobbling.

He says that there had been a phone call: that my mother had gone swimming that morning, that there had been a big wave, that the wave had knocked her over and that she had died. My mother has died. My mum was dead, is dead.

I see her stride into the water in her black Speedo swimsuit, a cap of white rubber roses high on her head and those swimming socks that kids wear on her incongruously tiny feet. I see her arms at her sides, hands turned outwards, always graceful, though she is heavy, always girlish though she is seventy-two. I see her lower herself into the water and start to swim, taking small, swift breaststrokes that somehow propel her forward. I imagine the water: clear, almost translucent, and warm. 'Ah, this is heavenly,' she says aloud to herself through the metallic-sounding suck of the retreating tide.

I see the wave she doesn't see, building behind her: huge, heavy, grit-filled. I see it crash down on my mother, I see her tumble, she looks frightened but as if it is a fright that she will recover from once she regains balance. Then I see her submerged and silent, hair floating above her and in her face, sand in her ears and her eyes, the muted sound of her own gasping breath. A gargled shout for help, unheard. No one knows that she is dying, has died. Under water it is still secret, still unknown and therefore still not true. Then up, ears pop, exposure and panic and shouting. 'Help!' 'Get her out!'

I can't imagine her face – I can't imagine it as not awake and not asleep, where there was always a flickering behind her lids, a twitch around her lips, a sense that she would wake again at any moment. Her swimsuit is shiny wet and bulging, her white hair made dark with the drenching. On the beach there are frantic attempts at resuscitation, people gather around her, kneel beside her, others run. But this is so far away from us. It is still a secret – an unseen, unheard thing. Far, far away from Bray, from me, from Charlie, from Nipey. It is unable yet to hurt us. Far away from Lifestyle Sports in Dundrum where my sister is shopping for runners. Her phone rings. It is our aunt. She has some news that she needs to rid herself of, and she just says it out straight. My sister says, 'No, no, no, no, no.'

*

I have a freeing, floating feeling as Charlie drives us through Bray high street on our way to my sister's home in Dundrum. My sister, a nurse, the practical one and now, abruptly an orphan, is the person my three other siblings and I gravitate to. I feel an odd sense of lightness, of relief. My mother is dead and nothing else matters – not work, not money, not friends, not worries – normal life is suspended, has stopped.

My eleven-year-old niece sits on the bottom stair and howls; my sister holds her. The front door is open as people come and go. I watch my big brother walk up the front drive, smiling his Mum-like smile, the one she would use before imparting any bad news. He is wearing a duffel coat that makes him look like a schoolboy and more vulnerable than I need him to be.

Lately, Mum had begun to pause on uphill walks, but she would never say she found them hard. She would simply stop, put her hands on her hips, lean slightly back on her feet, gaze out at the view and make some comment about it, until she felt able to continue. She liked to keep moving, she was no good at being still. Even when she was sitting at a dinner party or lecture (she still went to college, still got degrees) she would swing her legs below the table or desk. She was only five foot two, though she always seemed taller, and her feet never quite touched the ground.

She was cleaning out a kitchen cupboard when she told me that her blood pressure was a little high. She made a clatter with saucepans to drown out my questions and concern. She hated me worrying about her health. She was going on holidays, she was walking every day to keep fit, she was perfectly fine. She busied herself with her packing in the days leading up to her trip, taking pride in how efficiently she used limited space by rolling up all her outfits. The clothes she bought these days were selected not for their style or even for their colour, though she always knew what suited her, but for their un-creasability and comfort. Her suitcases were lightweight too, all her cosmetics travel-sized and already transferred into a see-through bag many days before departure, her travel documents arranged in a coloured wallet on the kitchen table beside envelopes for the gardener and the cleaner.

On the night before she left we all saw her to say goodbye. 'But you said you had a surprise for me,' her youngest grandchild complained as we were leaving. Of course, she'd almost forgotten. Mum trotted upstairs, humming tunelessly as she went, and returned with a small, big-eyed, toy Dalmatian dog for Nipey. She stood at the front door and waved at us; we waved back at her from the gate.

*

The next day, my sister collects me and the Nipe, and we all gather again, this time at my eldest brother's house in Rathmines. There is too much food on the kitchen table and more is continually being delivered to the door in cling film and tinfoil by neighbours. None of us can eat. We oscillate between normal and devastated, there are even moments of laughter. Texts ping into our phones every few seconds. Because Mum has died so far away, bringing her home is complicated. We contact embassies, ambassadors, honorary consuls, undertakers, check that her travel insurance will cover the repatriation of the body. Mum has a long final trip to take. First she is put on board a ship called *Legend*, later she is transported to the harbour, and from there to the cemetery of San Cristóbal. Another brother, the second eldest, who lives in the States, will travel from Boston to Ecuador to meet her, from there he will bring her back home. The youngest will catch the first plane he can from Washington, DC.

Charlie is not here yet but he is on his way. He is going to collect us and bring us home. I am lying under a duvet in the sitting room by the fire. The children are watching a movie beside me, unsettled by their suddenly rule-free lives: yes to more chocolate, we say, distracted, yes to staying up till ten.

When I answer the phone to Charlie I hear a long sigh and my stomach lurches.

'What's wrong?'

'Jesus, I've been driving around Dublin for hours. I don't know where the fuck I am.'

'Charlie, calm down. Where do you think you're near?'

'Down in the docks. I'm down in the bloody docks.'

The docks are nowhere close to my brother's home in Rathmines, which he has visited a dozen times. Advice is pointless when he is this angry – with himself for getting lost again, with me for asking to be collected, with my mum for up and dying, with my brother for living in fucking Rathmines.

I'm about to suggest that he ask for directions when he says he's going home and that he doesn't care how we get there. He hangs up. I curl into the foetal position, close my eyes. Why is he shouting at me when my mum has just died? Why is he looking for my attention when he should be looking after me and Nipey? Why is he being so useless and so selfish? Why the hell can't he find his way around Dublin any more?

When I get back later that night, in a taxi, my child asleep on my knee, I feel full of self-righteousness and determined not to forgive or even speak to Charlie. I settle the Nipe and go straight to bed. Charlie comes in; he is crying. He kneels on the floor beside me. He takes my hands in his, he says he is extremely sorry, that he loves me deeply.

'There's a badness in me,' he says, as he's said before. 'I got it from my father. You know that I adore you, don't you? I miss her too. I want to help you. I don't understand what happened.'

*

In the coffin at the funeral home there is a cross woman with heavy foundation and a downturned mouth. She is in my mother's clothes – the ones my sister and I had chosen for her – a long knitted purple cardigan with a white square pattern along the front and around the cuffs, black trousers, a pink blouse and a pearl necklace. But the necklace isn't where it should be. The front of it is tight around the woman's neck and the rest has fallen down the side of her body.

'That's not Mum,' I say aloud, and for a moment it really isn't and there is rush of adrenaline through me. They've got the wrong person. I need to see the big toe on her left foot where an ingrown nail had been removed many years earlier, but I can't bring myself to look at her feet – we'd chosen slippers rather than shoes to keep them warm. So I look away and try to focus instead on the painting that's on an easel beside the coffin. The portrait, a birthday gift from my big brother, who knew my mother would love to sit for an artist and chat to him as he worked, captured her in a way that no photograph ever did. In photos she often appeared out of focus, blurred, as if she was on her way to somewhere, or addled, the slight turn in her eye more evident than it was in real life. The brother who had travelled home with her body, the one Mum used to call 'the Bear', was the only one of us who had chosen not to see her dead; he wanted to remember her as she'd been. He is in the room with us but he keeps his head bowed. When they put the lid on the coffin, his bottom lip trembles and seeing this makes me start to cry again.

*

I see crowds of mourners standing in the forecourt of Donnybrook church, waiting for us to arrive. Inside, it is completely full, every pew taken, people standing at the rear. It's the fullest I've ever seen it. It makes me feel so proud of my mother but also weak with grief.

One of the undertakers stumbles with her coffin as he tries to rest it on the stand by the altar. Please, please don't drop her. Please don't be careless with something that requires so much care. Please no one make fun of my mum.

At the end of the service, I hold my little girl's hand as we walk towards the grey light of the opened church doors and the choir sings Fauré's 'In Paradisum'. I don't know where Charlie is – behind us or ahead – and I don't remember him beside us during the service though I know that he must have been. Last night after the removal of the coffin from the funeral home to the church, when there had been a gathering of neighbours and old friends back at my mother's house, he had asked me twice when we could go home because, he said, he was bored.

The light I imagine around my mum is golden. People bow their heads as we pass, bless themselves, feel in their pockets for tissues. So many of them are old and frail with limps and sticks and seem much closer to death than my mother. She had so many trips still to take. It was a beautiful way to go, everyone says, a beautiful death. And she always loved swimming, always loved the sea. I imagine her now, but as a young girl again, swimming at night in the inky still water of Bantry Bay towards the lantern-lit rowboat where her parents waited for her.

*

'Watch me, Mum,' my four-year-old says, bobbing below me in the water, her bright eyes fixed on mine to make sure she has my attention, her tiny fingers gripping the pool's edge. She takes a big breath, puts her thumb and finger over her nose and ducks under the water. Up she comes seconds later, her wet, perfectly round face beaming under an electric-blue cap.

'That was brilliant!' I say, bending towards her, a pair of blue plastic covers on my shoes.

'No, Mum, that wasn't it,' she replies, her little eyebrows arched. 'I can do it really goodly. Watch me again.'

It is the 25th of June, 2013. The doctors hadn't wanted to discharge me. They said I'd lost too much blood. I was weak, sore and grieving for the baby I had delivered and said goodbye to just the day before, but I was yearning to see the one who was still here, whose strong little heart was thumping below me now, solid legs kick, kick, kicking in the water.

My sister had collected me from the hospital and had driven me out to the swimming gala. I'd told Charlie to meet us there; it was close to our home in Bray. He isn't here when we arrive – all the children were brought directly to the pool by the Montessori bus – and I only become aware of him when the Nipe shouts at him to watch her too. I wave over and am about to make my way towards him when I see that he is scowling. I turn back to face the pool, try to locate my child in the water to distract myself from tears. Whatever the problem is, I am not strong enough to face it. Not today. Another father steps forward and offers me a seat. The other parents all know about the baby and are keeping a hushed and respectful distance.

I never wanted only one child. I'd grown up in a chaotic family of five, and the support of my siblings after my mother's death a year and a half earlier made me determined to try again. This was an IVF pregnancy that had taken a long time to achieve – I was now forty-four years old. I had a large early bleed and thought I had lost the baby, but her tiny heart, a blurry white dot on a black-and-white screen, was still pulsing away. When it happened again a couple of weeks later, I was told that I had a subchorionic haematoma (an accumulation of blood between the uterus and the placenta), that I needed strict bed rest and that I could lose the baby at any time.

Though I was confined to bed, the bleeding continued and a decision was made to admit me to hospital where I would spend a further month. It was very difficult to be separated from my daughter but Charlie was managing remarkably well without me – I resolved to help him less when I got home, to encourage his independence. He had become increasingly reliant on me since my mother's death, and I resented this dependence. He seemed less and less able to do things for himself, which I took for laziness and apathy. I was highly irritated by his behaviour and had long since given up expecting him to do anything with me. A second child was perhaps a mistake given how much we now argued, but I didn't want the Nipe to grow up on her own.

Twice when she'd arrived to visit – pushing with her dad to help open the heavy door to my room – she had bounded into my arms in tights but missing her skirt. He was just being a man, I told myself. The Nipe, quite fond of telling tales and getting others into trouble, whispered that her dad had forgotten her pizza in the oven one evening and it had burned. She giggled about him putting her in the bath with her socks still on and told me quite proudly that she had had to show him how to find my hospital room. Charlie visited once a week and generally didn't phone in between, but I accepted this; he wasn't used to minding his daughter full time, and I couldn't allow myself to worry about her when I was so focused on keeping the baby alive. It was a quiet battle being fought by the two of us, mother and unborn child; her survival was all I thought of each time I went to the bathroom, each time I flushed and saw blood.

I became happily institutionalized, with particular things I did at particular times of the day. Bed-bound as I was, my sense of hearing became more acute and soon I could differentiate between the sounds of the blood-pressure monitors, the dinner trolley, babies' cots and even the different walks: midwives – rapid and soft-shoed; consultants – noisier, purposeful; mothers in labour – a slow trudge with occasional pauses.

On a day when I'd got bad news about my baby – a blood test suggested that even if she made it, she might have serious health problems – I sat cross-legged on my bed in the dark and sobbed: the sort of sobbing that comes from your stomach, so natural as a child but physically painful as a grown-up. A midwife I'd never met before – dark-haired, large, from the country – sat on the side of my bed. 'You'll be OK, pet,' she said, sounding like my mum. Then she rubbed her hand along my leg, just as Mum would have done. 'You'll be OK, pet.' How those four words used to irritate me, so blasé, meaningless, offering no practical advice, no sign that she was taking my circumstances seriously. But that night they comforted me like no other words ever had, aside from the ones she said as she got up from my bed, again like the ghost of my mother. 'How about a nice cup of hot milk?' Not Valium, not Xanax, not two paracetamol or peppermint water, not even tea, but a nice cup of hot milk. And after my cup of hot milk she tucked waffle blankets around me, and I and my tiny, worn-out little fighter slept soundly.

'Am I not going to have a little sister?' our daughter asked on the day they couldn't find a heartbeat. When the baby gave up the fight it wasn't dramatic or violent, with sudden pains and bright blood on the bathroom floor, as had happened so many times in the seventeen weeks she'd been inside me. Each time I'd tell myself that she had gone, but each time there her tiny heart would be on the screen, beating impossibly on. When she left it was silent. She just curled up, cut off, shut down. Now I think I felt her leave; something made me lie down on the day her heart stopped beating, a sudden internal change took my energy away, made me feel overwhelmingly lost.

She fitted in the palm of the midwife's hand; her miniature legs dangled over its edge. 'Does she look like a baby?' I heard myself ask several times, and then I stopped asking that question. It wasn't fair of me to demand that my baby look baby-like when she had done so much just to try and stay alive. The midwife laid her down on a bed of cotton wool, lifted her into a small plastic container and handed her over to me.

Matchstick Man

Charlie inched forwards; both of us were frightened.

We looked down together at a tiny, perfect human being – everything was there and where it should have been: eyes, nostrils, lips. Her lifeless arms were crossed over her minute yet somehow swollen belly. A thick vein was visible beneath the still-warm skin of her head; it ran from the top of her forehead to just above her closed eyes. It made her look distressed. We didn't know what to do – it was torture to hold her and torture to hand her away. It was all warped, all wrong – mother and father with their newborn but their newborn was born too soon, born but dead, our baby but gone. They called her by the name we gave her, Lucia, they encouraged us to spend time with her, they could not have been any kinder. My sister said two of the nurses cried.

That night, another midwife made me a snack of cream crackers and cheese. I was still woozy with grief and from the general anaesthetic and she told me to stay lying down. I lay still and listened to her lick her thumb as she spread butter on each cracker, as though she were making a small meal for herself.

They hugged me – the dinner ladies, the domestics, the midwives, the consultants, the pastoral care workers – they held my hand, they sat with me, they prayed. *C'è sempre un perché*, there is always a reason, the lovely Italian nun told me – she had sought me out in the cafeteria when she heard that our baby hadn't made it. *C'è sempre un perché.*

We asked the Nipe if she would like to put anything in the shoe-box-sized coffin that Lucia would be buried in. She carefully selected some toys: a tiny white rabbit, a plastic bracelet, a doll's blanket to put over her. Later that morning she took them all back out – she didn't want her toys buried in the ground where she could never play with them, and she had already given Granny her ballet shoes.

*

It's the swimming gala finale. The children have been practising this part for weeks. They line up poolside like a row of pot-bellied little ducks. The Nipe is third, the boy in front of her needs the loo, the girl behind keeps shunting her forward. She searches for me in the crowd, folds her arms, shakes her head, mouths that she's not doing it. I make reassuring gestures, give her two thumbs up. She has never jumped in by herself before; like her mother, she is physically cautious.

I go to stand beside her dad. 'It's nearly over,' I say.

'Why did you drag me out to this fucking thing?'

'We promised her we'd be here.'

There's only one ahead of her now. He cannonballs in, soaks everyone. She seeks us out, waits to see if we are watching. I wave over.

'Fucking waste of my time.' He peels the blue covers off his shoes.

She edges slowly, slowly forward, her arms straight out in front of her, her focus on her teacher in the water, whose own arms are outstretched to catch her. Nipey hesitates, starts to whimper.

'I'm going to wait in the car,' Charlie says and strides to the door, which he cannot open.

The Nipe steps off the edge.

'Bastard!' he roars, trying again to pull the door that he needs to push.

She leaps into the air, curls her legs under her, dive-bombs into the water.

6

I'm lying on my stomach on the kitchen floor, over at the worn patch by the sink. The floorboards complain as I lean on them and stretch my arm into the dark space beneath the cabinets where dust and missing things accumulate. I feel blindly about for the front-door key. It's the last one we have, and I've already checked the lock, where Charlie sometimes leaves it when he lets himself in after a walk. I don't like being down here; I'm nervous of what I might find. When I opened the kitchen door the other evening, a small black creature darted from the bin to beneath the fridge: a mouse, or maybe a baby rat – our neighbours found a dead one in their cellar last week. I don't want to meet a baby rat or the rat bait that's on a saucer somewhere under here too. I pull out a Lego man covered in sticky black gunk, a chewed tennis ball, but no key.

I pick dog hair from my tongue and move to get up; an exposed nail on a board clings to my shirt and causes a small tear. I curse and look at the kitchen clock. The big hand is stuck and juddering behind the small one; it's eternally a quarter past three. I'm unsure of the actual time, but I know that I should have set off for the library long before now and that all the seats in the quiet room will be occupied. The students who trail in and out – restless, flirting, bored – are less distracting than Charlie on one of his searches: for his glasses, keys, wallet, phone, sometimes so frustrated when these objects elude him that he'll shout and break things, and I will have to stop what I'm doing and go to him. Or I'll find him standing at the top of the stairs, trying to remember why he climbed them seconds earlier with such purpose. Sometimes he'll come into whatever room I'm in and begin to tell me something. Then he'll pause and look at me for help, his mouth slightly open, his eyes full of worry. 'Sorry, it's gone,' he'll say as he goes back out, closing the door as quietly as he can so as not to disturb me further.

It's September 2013, four months after Lucia's birth and death. The Nipe and I had travelled alone to Italy the previous month to join some of my family there for a holiday – a happy thing for us both after all the sadness. Despite my pleading, Charlie had refused to come with us. He said the mosquitos would be biting; that he disliked the two untidy apartments jointly owned by my four siblings and me since our mother's death. I visited the baby's grave in the Angels plot of Glasnevin Cemetery a couple of times on my own, but the pain was still too raw – the teddies and brightly coloured plastic windmills too much to bear – and the long drive on the M50 through blinding tears too precarious to attempt regularly. A post-mortem said that she had died not because of any genetic abnormality but because the umbilical cord had become hypercoiled and had cut off the blood supply between us.

We both grieve for our baby, but privately, in different rooms. And we still begin each day together, after I have left the Nipe at her Montessori pre-school, with a walk along Bray seafront in the milky early light, down as far as the old hotel, stumbling over stones as we pick our way to the water's edge, where Blue waits, upright and alert, eyes locked on the ball in Charlie's hand. Home again and after a quick coffee I'll kiss Charlie goodbye on the forehead as I leave for the library. He'll look at me, forlorn. 'No, don't go,' he'll plead, wrapping his arms around me. 'Let's get back into bed for a bit.' It hurts him that I want to be away from him. He's the same when I say I'm meeting a friend for dinner or that I'm going for a bath; he's just happier when we're together on our own. 'I have to work,' I tell him, irritated, forcing myself free. 'We have to work, it's the middle of the working week.'

There's an unstable stack of upturned plates and bowls on the draining board and an assortment of sudsy cutlery. Charlie has stopped using the dishwasher; he prefers to wash things by hand these days, standing happy and quiet by the sink in his plaid pyjama bottoms, stopping only to slap off the radio if it gets too noisy or if he hears that Harvey Norman ad he hates.

I start to put away the dishes, but they still feel sticky with grease – a bit of last night's pizza is stuck between the prongs of a fork, traces of muesli line the rim of a bowl. For Christ's sake, I say aloud, tossing one, two, three dirty knives back into the sink. He has also begun lately to spend a lot of time ironing. Often when I get home in the evenings and call his name, I can tell from the direction of his reply that he isn't upstairs where I want him to be – absorbed in his work – but down in the utility room, bent over the ironing board. 'Ach, there you are, sweetie,' he'll say, resting the iron on its back and sliding out from behind the board to embrace me. And then: 'I haven't stopped, honestly,' in a slightly effeminate way, tilting his head in the direction of a pile of beautifully pressed towels and sheets. 'I do still make you happy, don't I?' he'll ask when I don't seem grateful. I know he does these things to be useful, to try to keep me content, to try and make some order of our increasingly disordered lives, but I worry that he is no longer painting.

On sunny days he'll set up a lounger in the back garden, pull off his vest and work on his tan, followed, perhaps, by a few hours of gardening, but most often he'll simply go back to bed. I tease him that his favourite position these days is horizontal. This amuses him. 'I'm a hard man. Hard in my underpants, hard to get up in the morning,' he'll say, laughing and waiting for me to laugh along like I used to. When he doesn't receive any softness he'll force himself upright. 'God almighty, I never get a break,' he'll say as he fumbles for his glasses on the bedside table. He'll tut at me for my bossiness, then take my hands in his and pull me close to him. 'I do love it when you barge me.'

Once a week he'll set off for the high street to buy paints and to have an argument with his bank: he'll yell at them that their useless fecking ATM still isn't working, thump his fist on it and kick the wall around it because he can no longer make sense of the information on the screen. 'And why do you keep changing my fucking PIN number?' he'll roar through the window, because he's forgotten the four digits he has always used. Customers inch away; cashiers shift in their seats, shoot glances at each other. Then he'll demand to know why they keep sending him cards that don't work – he doesn't understand that he can't withdraw money when all of his accounts are overdrawn. He'll return home, furious and without any paints, but with some bit of religious iconography or a china pig from the Vincent de Paul charity shop on the Quinnsboro Road and a story of some poor elderly woman or injured animal he helped along the way. Always empathetic, even when angry, always vigilant and watchful and curious – craning his long neck and turning his bald head in a cartoonish way to peer over the high wall of someone's garden. 'Good God,' he'll say if he notices the enormous backside of some unfortunate passerby, and he'll hold brief conversations with each dog he encounters and its owner, every industrious cat.

An unfinished painting has been resting on his easel for months. It's of the baby, Swee'Pea, from the Popeye cartoons. The baby's body in its red sleepsuit is complete but its face is just a round cream shape waiting for features. Charlie's chickens have lately been faceless too, or sometimes two-faced: two perfect beaks, one shadowing the other. At Halloween, with great difficulty, he carves a pumpkin – and gives it two sets of eyes but no nose. The Nipe sees that this is wrong, but she doesn't want to hurt her dad. She doesn't want to put a candle in it either. We find a discreet home for it in the back garden, where it slowly rots and caves in on itself. His last show, with his new gallery, the Peppercanister in Dublin, had been disappointing. He had to prepare for it while I was in hospital and he was minding the Nipe, and he only produced half a dozen new pieces – the rest he'd cobbled together from old works that had been stacked against the wall in his studio for several years or hung about our home. The resulting collection was disjointed and confusing. Only three paintings sold on his opening night, out of a possible twenty. He tried to be brave and philosophical about it, but I saw the hurt on his face. It was just the opening night, we told each other, the show would run for a further two weeks; but nothing more sold, and I knew it would take him time to rebuild his confidence. 'I'm working up to it,' he says whenever I ask when he might begin painting again.

At breakfast each morning, only getting out of bed when I've returned from delivering our child to Montessori, he sinks his teeth into a slice of Marks and Spencer's ciabatta bread, toasted and dripping with butter. I have to turn away or subtly cup my hands over my ears to dull the satisfied sound he makes as he eats, my mind full of irritation, resentment and questions, feeling ashamed of my meanness but angrily justified too: what will you eat when my money runs out? Why am I having to do it all on my own? Why won't you teach students at home once a week? I would do up fliers, I would distribute them, I would bring the students if you were willing to teach them. Why won't you apply for the art teacher vacancy in the local primary school? Why haven't you made any provisions for getting older? Why did you cash in your pension from NCAD to travel around India? Why aren't you trying to help support our child? I fire all of this at him silently, though I know he knows what I'm thinking. He blames the recession, the collapse of the Celtic Tiger, for taking away all his money and his motivation. He blames the bastards in the bank.

Still looking for the missing key, I search the dining room next. It's cold in here; the dark cabinets which had once seemed so right for the room are now oppressive, closing in on me and concealing things that we need. The mahogany table in its centre is as shiny and blemish-free as when we bought it seven years ago, when we still had optimistic plans for dinner parties, lists of potential guests and what vegetarian food we might feed them. But there was always some reason why the parties didn't happen, and the table has never been used; its leather seats are still perfect and plump, without the flattened imprint of wear or damage from rowdy, memorable nights.

There's a large cupboard opposite where I'm standing, one that Charlie had shipped home from India many years earlier. It's such a hulk that it entirely blocks the stained-glass window behind and it seems now to be listing to the right, as though the ground beneath is subsiding under its weight, as though it has given up trying to look its best now that it no longer needs to, now that we've decided to sell. The bank still owns more than half this house and we can no longer afford to pay them back. We are trying to live off my two-book deal but are almost at the end of it, my second book yet to be published – and this house was always too large for a family with just one child, and unmanageable given Charlie's tendency to hoard, and mine to hide chaos behind closed doors.

We spend whole weekends cleaning to prepare for viewings, our child silenced by the TV screen. We pull fresh duvet covers over grubby ones, pick dog dirt from the garden, light vanilla-scented candles, hoover carpets, build fires, put opera on the stereo, conceal the peeling enamel base of the bath tub with rubber ducks and foam alphabet letters. Charlie hides his human skulls and shunts the clay statue of Sister Scholastica deep into the mossy wet undergrowth beneath the mimosa tree that overhangs our garden from the Atlanta Home for the Elderly next door.

And then we wait in the park opposite the house, or in the car if it's raining, while strangers explore our home, unknown children test the swing in the garden or climb the ladder up to the Nipe's playhouse, seeing everything now as we once did. Before our first viewing, Charlie removed the elephant-grey cover from his Moto Guzzi, which he keeps in the driveway. Neighbours and passersby noticed it; this gave Charlie some pride – he answered their questions, reassessed its beauty himself. Now he's removed the cover for good but he no longer rides it – there's some sort of mechanical problem with it, he says. So it rusts, idle, sat on occasionally by a child on a play date, momentarily entertained before sliding back off with boredom. We decide to sell the Moto Guzzi too.

I open the Indian cupboard and lift out a heavy glass ashtray containing American coins, badges, safety pins – and reach for a wad of cards beneath it. I'm no longer looking for the missing key, now I'm in search of something else that's been bothering me. I sift through the cards till I find the one I want. Charlie gave it to me on my last birthday, when I turned forty-four, along with his usual gifts: a jumper from Topshop (always stylish, always grey, always the right size) and a couple of books – a slim volume of Emily Dickinson's poems and *The Poet and the Murderer* by Simon Worrall. I'd read the card while he'd hovered beside me in the kitchen, the Nipe on my knee, and had felt my stomach lurch:

Hapy Birthdy my darling, I stil love you to much.

There it was in the writing: the problem, now impossible to deny. I'd hugged him, thanked him, let the Nipe blow out my candles, spraying saliva over the chocolate icing. Later that day, I'd found the felt-tipped pen he'd used and had added the missing letters and put it back on the mantelpiece so I could pretend, to myself and anyone else who might open it, that everything was OK.

I can hear him upstairs now, going from room to room, still in search of the key. Neither of us is working and neither of us is earning, yet we are continuing to pay the local Montessori to mind our daughter all day.

Our home, the three of us as a family, is no longer functioning.

*

'That was such a broken thing,' Charlie says. We are sitting at the kitchen table; he slurps his tea while I huddle over mine, allow the steam to dampen my face – he has always been better able to tolerate hot liquids. When he puts the cup down, I can see that his hand is shaking. He is talking about Lucia, the baby we lost, about the pain of seeing her born dead.

'At least we have our Nipe. The wee bat,' he says, smiling at the thought of her – our beautiful, solid, perfect, healthy child, five doors down from us now. 'I can still see his face. The back of his head. The back of his head came off in my hand,' he says, holding his shaking fingers high and stiff in the air. He looks at them, wild-eyed, reimagining the horror and wanting me to imagine it with him, as though this was the first time he has described Michael's death to me. 'It never goes. His face. The poor wee thing.' He is remembering our tiny baby at birth and the bleeding head of the boy who had died in his arms. The two events, the two deaths, have somehow merged, become muddled, in Charlie's mind.

When I leave for the library an hour later, it's raining; the sort of rain that drenches you in seconds, pelting off the gutters, saturating the ferns and hydrangeas in the flowerbed, forming instant puddles on the porch and on the saddle of the old motorbike. I yell goodbye, make a dash for the car, holding my satchel over my head, yelping like a teenager. It's only as I'm reversing, at the gate and about to turn the wheel hard to the right to face towards Greystones, that I notice Charlie.

He is upstairs, at the sitting-room window, perched on the back of the sofa, his feet against the window ledge, watching me as I leave, watching the rain. Even in those few moments I can see that he is not simply crying, but howling so deeply, with such primal force and pain, that his face is entirely contorted. I know he will need to curl up with a hot-water bottle held to his stomach for the rest of the morning, to ease the spasms he gets when he is this distraught.

The Nipe found him trying to climb out through that same window on the night following a tiny funeral service we had for the baby at Glasnevin Cemetery: Charlie and me, a pastoral care worker from the hospital, the gravedigger, and Lucia in a small white box. The Nipe described what had happened to me the next day, sitting forward in her car seat, our eyes meeting in the overhead mirror as I drove. He had been thumping his fists against the glass – that was the sound that woke her – and when she came in she found him trying to prise the window open. She had taken him by the hand, told him he was just having a scary dream and had led him back to bed. 'I like taking care of Dada,' she said with an embarrassed smile, her one dimple indented.

We are all restless at night, each of us up and moving at different stages along the dark, carpeted landings, up and down the creaky stairs. Even the dog paces the hall to find a comfortable spot – the soft collapse of settling bones – and cries too loudly in his dreams, his claws digging into and marking the freshly varnished floors.

After Charlie's attempted escape I move back into our bedroom so that I can keep a closer eye on him. I've been sleeping in the spare room for many months – sex is a long-forgotten thing, sleep fitful and light, even with Xanax and ear plugs and meditations I've downloaded onto my phone. Charlie wakes another night that same week and gets up and dressed in the dark. I have a follow-up appointment at the maternity hospital early the next day and Charlie will be taking our child to Montessori.

'What are you doing?' I say, switching on the bedside light, squinting at the clock.

'I have to take the Nipe to school – have you forgotten about your appointment?'

'Charlie, it's 3 a.m. It's still night time.'

'Ach, Jesus,' he says, staring at the bedroom curtains for too long before getting back into bed, still dressed.

Unable to sleep, I take my phone from the table, plump a pillow behind my back and type a list of Charlie's symptoms into Google:

Short-term memory problems
Very tired
Very thin
Visual problems
Low mood
Upset stomach and flatulence

Then, one by one, I enter all the possible causes I can think of to find out what their symptoms might be:

Post-traumatic stress disorder?
Depression?
Stress?
Chemical imbalance?
Vegetarian diet?
Brain tumour?
Carbon-monoxide poisoning?
Exposure to high levels of radiation during a
     visit to Chernobyl?
Infection from dental implants?

I begin to keep notes of specific incidents. The time he put the car seat into the car upside down and tried to force our protesting daughter into it. The day he washed her hands in scalding water and was furious with her for screaming. The many, many times he had forgotten food in the oven. That evening when he put Nipey in the bath with her socks still on. The night he drove into oncoming traffic, swearing at the shock of headlights and horns and at me for grabbing the wheel. The morning he phoned me in the library to ask where the 'floor cleaner thing' was.

'You mean the mop?'

'No. You know, the floor cleaner thing.'

'The sweeping brush?'

'Jesus, no. The cleaner thing!'

'The hoover?'

'The hoover, the hoover. I can't find the fucking hoover. Where have you hidden it?'

One Saturday morning all three of us are in the bathroom together, grumpy from another disturbed night and the prospect of hours of cleaning ahead for an open viewing of our home that afternoon. The Nipe is brushing her teeth and Charlie is overseeing this activity while I scrub at a ring of grime round the bath.

Teeth done, she throws her brush into the basin, trots out of the room and back to her cartoons. Charlie shouts after her that she needs to rinse out her mouth. 'We never rinse out,' I say, flushed from standing up too swiftly, aware of how much this will annoy him. 'The dentist says it's better not to.'

'Bunkum!' he shouts, and calls her again, this time more aggressively. She reappears, Charlie takes the cruddy cup containing our toothbrushes, rests them on the sink edge, fills the cup with water and hands it to our child to drink. 'You can't give her that filthy thing,' I protest quietly. He grabs it back, flings it into the bath tub, its murky contents staining the wall. Then he calls us both fucking cunts.

Ten minutes later he comes down the stairs on all fours to see what it feels like to be a dog. The Nipe giggles – her love as unconditional as Mr Blue's.

I can't even look at Charlie. I walk past them in silence, through the kitchen and on out into the garden where I can breathe.

I pick up dog dirt, wandering around in my grey dressing gown. Someone is playing a trumpet – mournful and faltering – in the nursing home next door. Charlie often says that I should just toss him over the wall when the time comes, when he is too old and confused for us. I climb the ladder to the Nipe's wooden playhouse and crouch down, giant-like, in the damp and cobwebbed hut. He won't think to look for me here. I feel strongly at this moment that my daughter and I need to be free from this aggressive, lazy, unkind man. My heart has gone cold to him. We are a broken thing.

In the weeks that follow this outburst, I talk to my sister and a few close friends. I tell them I want to leave Charlie but that I'm worried he has become too dependent on me, that he won't manage on his own. I make an appointment to see our family doctor and set off on a bleak Friday evening. The Nipe screams to go with me, Charlie yanks her back indoors by the neck of her hooded top, incensed by her wailing and hurt by her rejection of him. I want to take her with me, I worry that she isn't safe when Charlie is this upset, but I don't want her to hear what I have to tell the doctor about her dad, about our family. The doctor sits back in his seat, tells me to take my time. I sob and shake for over an hour as I describe the situation at home. He listens, empathizes, says Charlie needs to be seen urgently. The doctor feels Charlie may be depressed and he wants him to take some memory tests.

There was one thing I missed in those dark last months before the sale of our home, despite my concern for Charlie and my increasingly close observation of him. I noticed that he was continuously removing and rehanging paintings around the walls of our home, but what I failed to see was that he had taken every one of his unsold paintings from the walls, and those stacked up in his studio, and had painted over each one of them in white.

*

'That's not good, is it?' Charlie says when the consultant at the Memory Clinic tells us that he has Alzheimer's disease. It is the 8th of April, 2014. He turns to me and puts his hand on my shoulder as though I'm the one who has been given the diagnosis. It's too hard to watch Charlie try to absorb these words. I look instead at the beige plastic chairs pushed under the Formica table, a large green folder, a brown envelope, the two men sitting opposite us: one black, one white. One a stranger, the other the husband of an old school friend of mine. Charlie lets go of my shoulder and joins his hands on his lap. I slip my hand between his. We both look down at his feet, at his Converse high-tops.

The two men try to reassure us, they tell Charlie that there are still many things that he can do, they tell him of all the support available to him, they tell him that there will be medication to slow the progression of the disease. Then they ask him to sit in the waiting room so that they can chat to me on my own. I don't want Charlie to be in that empty room with out-of-date magazines, the TV just below audible. I don't want him to be left alone to try and make sense of what has been said, or to know that we are discussing him in his absence.

But he leaves the room, and now, no longer needing to be brave, I break down. Without Charlie there, both doctors are more honest, less philosophical about the future. The smiling models on the glossy 'Dealing with Dementia' brochures I have been given do not fool me for one moment. This really is every bit as bleak and as bad as it sounds. I tell them that things are not good between the two of us, that I don't know how we will manage, that I can't stand the thought of all he will have to endure, that I am so worried about the impact all of this will have on our young child.

I cry openly as I drive us both home; beside me, Charlie is buoyant. Now he has a name for what is happening in his head, an excuse for all he has done wrong. He had endured six months of brain scans, memory tests, blood tests, weekly visits to a counsellor to help him with his depression, along with daily antidepressants. Now there would be no more need for investigations; we could slow everything down. I feel so close to him. I want to take care of him, I can't stand how frightened he must feel. I tell him again and again that he will not be facing all of this on his own.

Three days later he breaks down in the kitchen. 'I don't want to be the one on the seafront that everyone laughs at,' he says. I know we are both thinking of the chicken boy. Or the man who would stand at the bottom of the Seacliff Road in Bangor every morning, looking this way and that, hands joined behind his back, never going anywhere, just watching and waiting.

Charlie asks me not to tell anyone and I feel that I have betrayed him, as I have already confided in my family and close friends. He feels embarrassed by his illness, ashamed of it and very, very scared. I hold him, tell him that he will always be Charlie, that no one is laughing at him.

Inside I feel trapped; all I see ahead is a grey vortex of padded envelopes and doctors and social workers and blister packs, a great miserable weight of responsibility and guilt and anxiety, a downward spiral for Charlie that I must travel along too. I already feel that I am not doing enough for him but at the same time resentful for having to do so much, too much. There is no conceivable happy ending to this. I cannot now leave Charlie, no matter how deeply unhappy I have become. This is what our lives will be for the rest of Charlie's life, until he can no longer feed himself, until he forgets how to swallow, until everything that is Charlie is stripped away.

*

My second novel, *The Playground*, is published in September 2014. So many copies are pre-ordered that it is reprinted before the night of the launch. My editor is delighted, there is a large and supportive crowd and drinks back at the hotel we are staying in, the Nipe eating room-service chips and watching movies with a teenage babysitter, excited by our excitement and by being up so late. Charlie is proud and upright all evening, pretending to recognize everyone, losing his train of thought often but hiding or laughing off his mistakes.

I had joked to our neighbours that I hoped we'd have moved before my second novel was published as all of them were in it. This wasn't true, of course – though, like all writers of fiction, I create characters from observing the habits, appearances and traits of real people and then fusing them into something imaginary.

Shortly after my novel comes out, someone makes us an offer on our home. There's a sense of movement and change at last and it gives us a new and happier energy. At breakfast time a few weeks later, Mr Blue's heart-leaping bark tells us that someone is at the gate – Charlie goes to see, the Nipe skips after him and runs back through the hall into the kitchen moments later: 'There's a parcel for you, Mama!'

I grab it and take it with me in the car, toss it on the passenger seat along with the rest of my post and go for a walk up Killiney Hill with Mr Blue. Back in the car with a panting dog and mucky boots, I pick it up. The address is handwritten and there's no stamp. I turn it on its back to open it. Above the seal are the words 'Go back to Dalkey ASAP'. I have never yet lived in Dalkey, so this is clearly from someone who doesn't know me very well – but well enough to know where I live now and where I am hoping to move to.

I open the envelope. Inside is a copy of my second novel, its pages hacked from the spine and ripped into tiny pieces, thousands of jumbled-up words, the cover picture of a child on a swing, beheaded and sliced through the middle.

7

I career over speed bumps in Charlie's old Volvo, the queue of cars behind forcing me to go faster than I want. I don't trust my driving on this narrow, winding road, or the car which has lately begun to cut out without warning. I imagine the accident: the slam of a hand on a horn, the skid and smash of collision, the whack of my head on the windscreen. I'm collecting the Nipe from a play date at a house I've never been to before. I need to take the first right beyond the church, the spire of which I spot a fraction too late; I brake and swerve across the road. The driver behind revs his engine as soon as he's clear of me. I catch a flash of his furious arms in the air through the overhead mirror.

I'm addled, a word my mother used to describe herself when she had her children hanging off her, twenty guests on their way over for dinner and the buttery mix of failed profiteroles in the bin. It's early

Julia Kelly

November 2014, six months since Charlie's diagnosis.

A new family will be moving into our home in Bray in three weeks' time and we have yet to find somewhere else to live. I'm stiff and sore from shifting boxes and furniture, my hands dry and cut, nails broken. We have been trying for months to declutter, to sell or give away to charity belongings we no longer need, but the task is too large and overwhelming and some things, like baby clothes, are too hard to let go of. I can't sell my buggy and high chair to some fertile, optimistic woman whose straightforward life I imagine and resent. I've kept them since the Nipe was born, and I still see myself as having two children one day.

I know I've been impatient with Charlie while we've tried to pack up, sometimes unkind, asking for his help to move something and becoming immediately irritated if he looks confused or tries to carry it to the wrong place, or when he can't follow my rushed and garbled instructions. Several times I've told him to forget it, that I'll do it myself – leaving him redundant in the centre of an empty room. Since his diagnosis he has stopped pretending to understand, has stopped laughing off his mistakes. There has been a letting go and a gradual handing over of roles. Now I am in charge; when I wake each morning I feel that I am on duty, that I should put on a uniform and a badge. By evening I'm always crotchety and self-pitying – telling Charlie that I'm tired of doing everything on my own; that I wish I had someone to look after me; knowing that he wants desperately to be needed and appreciated but is no longer up to a task as disorientating to his newly diseased brain as moving house. He has generally tried to stay out of my way, often retreating quietly back to bed.

Occasionally he tries to lighten things by wearing his iguana mask around the house or his silly Afro wig. Distracted while emptying out a chest of drawers the other morning, he tried on his father's old Orange Order sash, then the sleeveless leather jacket he wore in his twenties. He came downstairs to model it for me and Nipey, his white, pin-thin arms on his hips. He doesn't want to leave our home, or Bray, and he no longer understands that we have no choice but to sell. He also doesn't want to be without any of his things. And though we will never again have a home that could fit all his furniture, his possessions are tied so tightly to Charlie's identity that it feels cruel to get rid of any of them.

'Don't make the mistake of paying to store things you'll never need again,' the removal man advised when he dropped round to assess the job the other evening. The scene felt old-fashioned: the two of us standing there in the dark hall; the removal man in brown slacks and a taupe sweater, me wearing washing-up gloves and an apron. He remembered my mother, he said, with a shake of his head. He had moved her to her new home several years before her death. He seemed jaded, as if he'd seen lives unravel too often.

Everyone is telling me what to do – friends, social workers, doctors, family – and everyone has differing advice. My brother the economist in the States says we shouldn't buy another house. He'd said the same thing last time, when we weren't listening and went ahead and bought one we could never afford. My other siblings are adamant that I should buy something, even a small apartment, so that when I'm broke between book deals we will still have somewhere to live.

One idea I've considered is to buy a small house with a garage that I could turn into a granny flat for Charlie, so that he would be away from the pressures that he had started to find intolerable, but the family would still be intact. There is now an underlying tension whenever the three of us are together. We all know that happy, calm moments are transient, and will be shattered, inevitably, by a tickle too far, glasses slipping unseen down the side of the sofa, the Nipe getting giddy or bored. Charlie still likes to play his music loud, but there is a rhythm, a predictability to this sort of noise: lyrics and melodies that have endured in his mind. They don't irritate him the way the high energy and erratic movements of an active child do. He puts his hands over his ears at the slightest whine or cry and roars at me to take her away, that he can't be around 'the little brat'. Then I'll shout at him for being so mean and the Nipe will sit silent at the kitchen table, creating cards with messages like 'I love you so much Dada' or 'I'm sooooo sorry Dad', unsure of what it is she has done wrong.

*

As I negotiate the potholed laneway of Shanganagh Terrace and begin to look for the Nipe's friend's house, I realize that I've been here before. Charlie drove me down this lane seven or eight years ago, when we were looking for a house to buy. We could never have afforded a home in this area – near the golden coast of Killiney – but reality was irrelevant to us back then. What I recognize first is the quirky layout: the houses – a pleasantly chaotic mix of styles, some Victorian villas, some detached red-bricks, some Georgian – have small front gardens, with a larger plot of land opposite each one, intersected by the lane-way. Some of the gardens are well tended: freshly cut grass, cleanly edged; cream roses; blue hydrangeas; neat stacks of brambles for bonfires. Others are over-grown, with cracked terracotta pots on their sides, wilting plants in ancient greenhouses with broken windows. Beyond the gardens is a tangle of greenery and the suggestion of further habitats: weather vanes, pitched roofs, smoking chimneys.

A lame, grey-faced Labrador pit-pats in front of the car as I try to find the house where my daughter's friend from her new school lives. She has started at a small Church of Ireland national school near Bull-och Harbour in Dalkey. It means a long and fast drive from Bray each morning, but I chose it because I know we'll be leaving Bray soon and hope to move nearer to Dublin and closer to my family. I have friends in the area, a support group of sorts, and the classes at this school are small – there are only twelve in our daughter's year. Within weeks she has learned the name of every child in the building, her teachers are kind and understanding of her dad's condition and the parents are warm and inclusive, with regular invitations to play dates and parties.

I've been told I can't miss the house. It's a large, semi-detached Victorian lodge, its yellow painted exterior chipped and peeling. An Egyptian god and goddess bearing lamps flank the base of the steps, and in the garden the grass is scattered with children's scooters and toys, discarded jumpers, empty crisp packets. I park in a gravel area opposite – here there is no second garden but a patio of sorts, with a white cast-iron table and chairs and a disused Renaissance-style fountain. The Labrador, still ahead of me, cocks her leg and pees on a half-empty sack of cement.

I'm looking for the bell when the door is opened by a barefoot teenage girl with auburn hair down to her waist and a rabbit in her arms. She smiles shyly at me, says excuse me, runs down the steps, releases the rabbit into a wire cage in the front garden and goes on out into the laneway. I flatten myself against the door frame as half a dozen more kids spill out, followed by a guinea pig. They're excited and focused, as if a game has just been agreed, someone chosen to be 'on' – all of them are also barefoot or in dirty socks. The Nipe is the last child to appear. She's hurrying too, but physically cautious; she keeps one hand on the banister and her eyes on her feet as she goes. Safely down, she looks ahead and is disgusted to see me. 'We didn't even have time to play screaming angel!' She dissolves into tears and slumps down on the bottom stair. I tell her ten more minutes. 'You're the best mum in the whole universe even if we were on different planets,' she says as she hugs my legs.

We sit on the front steps, the other mother and I, half-watching the children, who are now having a water fight despite the November chill. They're at that level of high excitement which is only seconds away from hysterical crying. The Labrador has her bum in the air, snout down, trying to get access to the rabbit, which is thumping its paws to deter her. 'How are you today, Val?' the mum shouts over to a man in his fifties, rooting for something in a small shed beside the fountain. 'Bloody marvellous!' he replies, though he looks creased and vague, as if he has just woken from a nap. He steps around us, a heavy picture frame in his arms, and disappears indoors. The mother tells me that he's the landlord, that he lives in the flat beneath her, her husband, four children, a guinea pig and a hamster – and there's a poet living at the back in a sort of annexe.

'I love every season at Shanganagh Terrace,' she says. She tells me about the fireworks they'd had on Halloween night, about the Christmas parties to come and of summer evenings sitting out on the steps, sharing bottles of wine with their neighbours. This seems such a cheerful, informal place to live compared to the stiffness and relative loneliness of our years in Bray.

I haven't found out who left that parcel on our doorstep. 'They could have done worse,' the guard said as he examined the shreds of my book before putting them in a plastic bag and sealing it. He asked if I could think of anyone who might hold a grudge against me. I couldn't, but it made me worry that the way I write – always from my own life – has caused someone so much hurt that they were driven to do such an aggressive thing, and I feel unnerved at the thought that we are being watched and hated by some unknown person. I worry for our safety; I don't want to spend another night in the house.

During our chat the mother mentions that the basement flat is currently vacant; before we leave I ask her if I could see it. We stand together in a small courtyard below a listing art deco street lamp, its base covered in blue duct tape, and peer in through stained-glass windows: dust dances in slants of sunlight above a parquet floor, the dark furniture – purples and plums – paintings and quirky statues remind me of Annaghmakerrig, and from where I'm standing I can see the kitchen beyond, with a pretty, French-looking, purple, green and white tiled floor. She tells me the place is available to rent and that Val is looking for very little – all that matters to him is that he likes his tenants. In that moment I can easily imagine the three of us living there.

I want the Nipe to experience some of the happy chaos of the childhood I'd had: egg fights and pillow fights and midnight feasts and pulling down our knickers to make our brothers get out of our room and cat pee on beanbags with their insides pulled out and pudding-bowl haircuts and unmatching socks and trips to 'Rats' Lane' with plastic buckets to get blackberries and climbing in bathroom windows in the middle of the night and standing on our brothers'

heads and them making us run around the large playing field behind our house before we were allowed to
have a piece of our mum's home-made coffee cake. I
want her childhood to be more carefree, less full of
anger and worry and stress. Lately, when she sees
that I'm starting to wobble, she takes my phone, finds
Bill Withers's 'Lovely Day' and encourages me to sing
along with her.

She caught me crying as we hurried into school
the other morning, up the cruelly cold path beside the
church.

'What's the matter, Mum?' She stopped and stood
looking at me.

'Nothing, I'm fine, let's go.'

'Mum, I've known you for nearly six years. I think
I know when you're upset.'

I said my sister had told me a sad story earlier, but
she knew I was really crying about Charlie. When she
had begun to ask why he was making so many mistakes, I'd told her that all brains get smaller as people
get older and that her dad's brain was just getting
smaller more quickly. She gets embarrassed when I
talk to her this way, too seriously, too attentive to her
reaction.

'It's fine, Mum. Why are you watching me? I don't mind that he forgets things. He's still funny,' she says, breaking into a smile at the very thought of his funniness. There is no higher compliment that she can pay him, no greater virtue to a five-year-old than being funny.

*

At the hospital Charlie is taken off to be weighed, like a small baby, while I am brought in to see the consultant. There are several uniformed staff in the room. I'm unsure of their roles and they keep their heads down, chew on their lips, periodically look up to eye me with concern. The consultant isn't sure whether Charlie's low mood is a symptom of his Alzheimer's or whether it is the knowledge of his illness that is causing his depression. The type of depression that is brought on by external events – the type the consultant thinks Charlie has – does not respond well to drugs.

Although he now struggles to get dressed – trying to squeeze his head into the arm of his sweater, removing it, laying it straight on the bed to see what goes where, then trying again and failing and calling himself a useless fucker – Charlie remains entirely lucid. He sees every error, he has a front-row seat to the deterioration of his mind.

Charlie is brought back into the room. I don't understand why the consultant feels that now is a good time to discuss this, but he says that I need to think ahead to when Charlie will have to go to a nursing home. Charlie's wearing his baseball cap, his leather jacket and his Converse trainers. His clothes don't go with 'nursing home' and the words don't register with him.

'Is it still safe for me to have sex with my girl-friend?' Charlie says, when the consultant, gathering his papers, asks if we have any more questions.

All eyes swivel to the ground. 'Can we have sex or am I contagious?' he says.

'Charlie,' I say, sounding embarrassed, but what I feel is pure pain. I hate that he has so little physical contact with anyone any more. I wish I could give him that sense of contentment, but I can't lie to myself and I don't want to confuse him further. We have talked many times of my wish to separate, but he seems to forget these chats and doggedly refers to me as his girlfriend. We still hug, he still likes to slip a hand under my thigh to 'wedge' me and I still let him kiss me on the lips and always will, but I can't do any more than that. 'I wish we could start again,' he says often, but he no longer waits for my response.

He is asked for a second time to sit in the waiting room, and I am brought in to see a social worker. Although all of this is about him, he spends so much time outside rooms that everyone else is in, discussing him. The social worker says I look exhausted. I tell her how things are for us at home. She listens, takes notes, her facial expression alternating between concern and alarm. I have told our story to so many people in recent months that I have become immune to the words and the impact they have on others.

She says she feels strongly that we need to live separately. I get the sense that she thinks this is what I want to hear. It is true that conditions at home are tough and miserable, but I don't know how the Nipe and I can leave. I can't abandon him when he is so vulnerable, and I can't stand the hurt that a split would cause to him and our child. So I try to reassure her that it is manageable. I backtrack, I play things down.

She is unconvinced and tells me several times that it is an urgent child-protection issue. For a few panicky minutes I worry that our daughter might be taken from us. 'You know your daughter can't go on living in that atmosphere,' she tells me gently. 'The situation you're describing is too threatening for a small child.'

'But I don't want to break up our family,' I say. 'And people will think I've left Charlie because he's sick.'

'You need to stop caring about what other people think. If you carry on as you are, your daughter will have two very unwell parents, and you cannot do that to her.'

I inhale deeply to stifle tears. The social worker says she's worried that I might have a breakdown. This makes me feel that I'm not coping, but also that I no longer have to pretend that I am. Everyone tells me that I am strong, but I am not strong; I have never felt weaker or more lost than I do right now. And like a child who receives pity when retelling some story of injustice, I find the social worker's empathy such a relief that I finally let go. Once I start crying, I can't stop. I am taken to a room upstairs where I sit on a seat beside a hand sanitizer. I don't know how long I'm there but someone must have paged my sister, who works in the adjoining hospital, because now she is kneeling beside me, holding my hands. Charlie is still in the waiting room. I know he will be unsettled, wondering where I am and confused because no one is telling him what's going on.

*

When I take Charlie to see Shanganagh Terrace a week later, it's no longer with the idea of the three of us living there together, but now as a possible new home for him and Mr Blue. The rent is low, it's less than five minutes' walk to the sea and the train station, close to the local shops and several of Charlie's old friends. He likes the area and immediately remembers it. Before we have even met Val, he is chatting to the elderly woman who lives next door and has befriended the old Labrador.

I keep things very vague with Val and the other residents – I don't tell any of them outright that Charlie has Alzheimer's. I simply say that he is becoming quite forgetful and that he needs some help with daily tasks. I struggle with this decision. I know it's dishonest and I worry that there may be an incident, but I feel this place is right for Charlie and I can imagine him being happy here. People get scared when they hear the word Alzheimer's, it's just better left unsaid until he is properly settled in.

So Charlie moves into the basement flat. We hang his favourite paintings around him, put Ted and Beanbag on his bed. Mr Blue settles in the sitting room beside the TV. My sister offers the Nipe and me a room at her house in Blackrock until Christmas. I will travel to Killiney to see Charlie twice daily, to care for him, and his grown-up daughter, Domino, who has just moved back from the States, will come out in the afternoons. Domino, Charlie's ex-wife Mariad and I become Charlie's support group. There is no formal agreement or discussion about it and there's no room for any awkwardness between us; we come together quite naturally. We are the three people closest to Charlie, and he is the focus of our attention. We are also allocated a carer by the Health Service who will come at lunchtime each day and stay with Charlie for two hours.

In a mood of practical optimism, Domino buys stickers in Eason's and we go around the flat together, labelling machines and switches. She writes careful instructions for her dad for how to operate the TV, how to work the CD player, and I label the fridge and the freezer. Charlie shadows us as we work, insisting that it isn't necessary, that he can figure these things

159

out for himself, but then he backs down and begins to make suggestions for labels that might help him.

Before we leave, he asks us if we could please write out instructions for how he can kill himself.

8

It's early evening when we arrive at Shanganagh Terrace, and it's getting dark. The Nipe waves up at the black silhouettes of children watching us from their bedroom window. She's been at swimming lessons and is in her pyjamas and slippers, her hair tied up in a sodden bun. She shouts things to the kids that they can't hear, but one by one their heads disappear and they thunder down the stairs to open the front door for her. I tell her she has one hour. This is a habit we have quickly fallen into: the Nipe plays with the children upstairs each evening while I spend time with Charlie in his flat below.

Everyone in the house has warmed to Charlie in the four months he's been living here, and he is often invited to join the rest of the household for dinner – he phoned me drunk the other night to say that they were all lying on the sitting-room floor, he wasn't sure why. Val gives Blue daily treats, and the kids spend happy hours throwing balls up and down the laneway for him. This set-up means I can visit Charlie on his own, without worrying that the Nipe will unwittingly cause a problem or that she might witness her dad in some form of distress.

This evening he is in high spirits. Bob Dylan is crooning from the stereo, the gas fire is alight. He wants to help me with the heavy bags of groceries I'm carrying through the hall. He always wants to physically unburden me. It bothers him if my handbag is too full or when I wear uncomfortable shoes. He tries to take one of the bags from my hand but we struggle with the exchange – he can't seem to see the handle, is unable to catch hold of it. I lower it to the floor so that it's easier for him to lift up, but he grabs the side of the bag instead, causing everything to fall out. 'Jesus,' he says. 'I'm a buck eejit.' I reassure him but I'm sure he hears me sigh as I bend down, stuff it all back in and hurry through the hall ahead of him.

He doesn't let my impatience upset him, and as I unpack he shadows me, still wanting to help. He tells me about the trip he and Domino took that day to the Alzheimer's Society centre in Blackrock. He describes a large room filled with people shuffling about and dithering, 'all half mad as I'll be soon,' he says. 'They're going to try and make a corner for me where I can paint. It's a very nice place and not too far from the sea.' To hear him sound so upbeat and appreciative makes me feel acutely sad. He had always been so interested in aesthetics, demanding attractive surroundings, a beautiful home, a pretty partner, an expensive car, a large studio. Now he is excited by the prospect of painting in the corner of a room in a centre for people with dementia.

At the start of our relationship I saw his interest in beauty as purely a part of his visual, observant and creative nature. It was only when we ran out of money and he continued to want these things around him that it irritated me, and then I began to resent what I saw as a materialistic and shallow attitude. Simple things make him happy now: the intense redness of a flower, the pattern of a night sky, walking along Killiney Beach, hot whiskeys, chocolate ice-cream.

We sit at the small kitchen table together; a Sylvanian badger peeps out between the leaves of some fake flowers between us. I put my hand on his. He tells me that he had a dream about us last night:

he dreamt that I was writing a book about him. I tell him that I *am* in fact writing about us, that this is all I can write about at the moment, as my mind is filled with thoughts of nothing else. I had had an idea for my third novel but when I sat down to begin it, I just couldn't concentrate, so I had started instead to make notes about Charlie and our lives. When I say all of this, he sits upright.

'Will you write a book about me?'

'About your illness? Would you like me to?'

'I want people to understand what's happened to me. Will you explain why it all went wrong, so they'll know it wasn't my fault? Will you put Arnold in?' he asks, recalling his childhood friend. 'And Michael Browne?' – the murdered boy. 'And when I worked in LA?' He is adamant that I must write the book, that he can help, and that he will give me lots of material.

Ever since his diagnosis I had been thinking that I should write down some of Charlie's childhood memories before they were gone from him, so that the Nipe would be able to read them when she's older. I also felt compelled to record what this illness had done to our relationship, and I wanted to tell the story of our years together and how things had come apart between us – perhaps as a form of self-defence, or a sort of therapy to help me work my way through it.

'But I'll have to tell our whole story, Charlie, I'll have to include the parts when you've been a pain in the ass. I'll have to be totally honest.' He smiles, pushes his chair back, winces at the screech it makes against the tiled floor, stands up and hugs me.

We hear them coming then; half a dozen children swarm in through the hall, led by the Nipe. They gather in the second bedroom; a low-ceilinged, windowless and permanently hot room (there's a radiator by the bed that can't be turned off). There's confusion over the ownership of this room, and it has already caused several arguments between the Nipe and her dad. We agreed to tell our daughter that it was her room so that she would always feel welcome in Charlie's home, but Charlie has since moved his paintings and other precious things in and he doesn't want any of it disturbed. I ask him to pretend it's hers even if it is not. He doesn't understand this. I tell him that he needs to at least try and act like a father for the small amount of time he spends with his daughter. As soon as I've said this I regret it; it's cruel of me. He often offers to mind the Nipe, but I always dismiss his help.

I can't tell him that he may no longer be left alone with his daughter – not even for ten minutes, one doctor told me.

There are now too many children in the place and their presence is unsettling Charlie. I realize that, much as he wants me to be here, I am also unsettling to him. I speak too fast, I move too swiftly, my thoughts flit from topic to topic, I am easily distracted and I do too many things at once. Charlie gets up and begins to move back and forth. He says he is looking for something, but he can't remember what. He gives up, creeps into the second bedroom and lets out a roar that makes all the children scream. Nipey laughs and looks at her friends with pride. She begs her dad to do it again. Then he remembers what it was he was looking for. He brings me into his bedroom. He tells me that he met a nice Italian man that afternoon, who stopped to ask him for directions as he and Blue were on their way down to the beach. The man had then given him a lift into Dalkey village; he even drove Charlie to the bank machine to help him to withdraw two hundred euros to buy some Italian leather goods. I'd heard about this con man on the radio, preying on vulnerable people and selling them fake leather coats.

'I thought this would do for your sister,' Charlie says, pulling an ugly brown leather jacket from a plastic bag and holding it up for me to see.

*

When I show Nipe the apartment I've found for us to rent, she puts her hand over her mouth in astonishment, her blue eyes bright as anything. Then she runs through the open-plan room. 'Is it really ours?' she asks again and again, jumping on the sofa, trying out the telescope, climbing up on to the window seat. I have the sense that she is putting this on somewhat, that she is playing up her happiness because she feels that I need her to be happy, but we had been living in my sister's since we moved out of Bray and she had talked all that time about having our own home again. It had been a difficult few months, sharing a bed, living out of suitcases, and with Charlie panicking and running away as he did, just days before Christmas.

The apartment is high on a hill, only a five-minute drive from Charlie's flat, with huge windows that face the sea. The Nipe gets so giddy that she wets herself and then has the most dramatic tantrum of her five years. She refuses to leave – we aren't moving in for another week – and I have to drag her out and carry her down the steps to the car while she kicks and screams and bites me.

For the first few months at the new apartment, I feel shaky and am overcome at night by a fear that I will become ill and that the Nipe will wake to find that I have collapsed. I put the numbers of my sister and two friends who live close by into my phone and show her how to find them. She senses my fear and then her own fears begin – she rejects her own bed and moves in to mine. Each night, curled up beside me, fighting sleep, she is full of anxiety and reasons to keep talking:

'I do like our new house, but I was happy when we were all together in the old house.'

I tell her that we couldn't afford to live in the old house any more.

'Why can't Dada and Mr Blue move into our new house?'

'It isn't big enough for Dada and Blue.'

'Can Dad and Mr Blue have a sleepover with us at least?'

'Maybe, now off to sleep.'

'Will you marry Dad some day?'

'No, that's not going to happen.'

'But will he always be my dad?'

'I promise he will always be your dad.'

She pauses, seeming satisfied with this. Then she says: 'So one day I might have a second dad, but Dad will always be my real dad?'

'That might happen one day, sweetie. How would you feel about having a second dad?'

'I don't mind so long as he tickles me.'

A day later, she meets me behind the sofa. I'm not sure what we're both doing there, but this is where we converge.

'If my new, second dad was really nice and fun and kind and tickled me when you were there but was mean to me when I was by myself, who would you believe?'

'Always you,' I say, feeling out of my depth and wondering whether she should see a counsellor.

For her sixth birthday, that February, I buy her a white labradoodle puppy. Nipey names the puppy Sunny and says that she is her little sister. The dog makes us both feel safer and helps our apartment feel more like a home. We fall into a chaotic sort of routine. I walk the Nipe and Sunny to school, pulled all the way by the puppy, the Nipe cautious on her scooter behind us, then it's home and into the car to drive to

Charlie's to get him up and give him his breakfast. A carer arrives mid-morning and Domino is there every afternoon. I return in the evening when I've collected the Nipe from the childminder's and drive too fast back over Killiney Hill to give Charlie his tea. Before I go after dinner I give him a Xanax – he's on three a day now – washed down with red wine and a Magnum ice-cream.

Leaving is often like something from the pantomime – as soon as I get one thing settled, another falls out of place. I'll get Blue out of the hatchback boot he has leapt into in the vain hope of a walk and put Sunny in, while trying to keep Charlie safely indoors and the Nipe in the car with me. Finally, Blue will be in his bed, Charlie on the sofa waiting for his second carer, who comes for an hour each evening, Sunny's white head will be visible in the car, but the Nipe will be missing. Back upstairs, one child asks another and I drag mine out protesting, secure her in her seat. The narrow and busy laneway requires endless reversing and turning and pulling over and waiting in order to get out of it. At home, once the Nipe is asleep, I will run myself a deep bath, lie with my head under the water, listen to my own breath.

'You take on too much. You need to slow down,' Charlie said to me the other day. It's true. I'm running on adrenaline, in a permanent hurry. He says I am always leaving and this is true too, I am. But Domino and I feel happy that, together, we are pulling this off. This precarious transition seems to be going smoothly, and Charlie is in buoyant form.

*

We are least at odds when we walk together, me always a few steps ahead because I want to get in shape. Charlie doesn't stride any more; he moves slowly now, with a new tentativeness and a vagueness in his eyes as he concentrates on the uneven ground beneath him.

He is quieter on our walks these days. When I say this to him I know he can hear the slight irritation in my voice. I want to have a conversation. I want him to notice things, as he always has done, I want him to stop calling Sunny 'he'. I correct him every time he gets it wrong, though I know it's unfair and unnecessary.

'You don't need this,' Charlie said to me the other day, suddenly upset. Meaning himself, his illness, Charlie and Alzheimer's disease. We had paused at the base of the hill to watch Sunny tumble on the grass with a young beagle. The fluid movement of their rolling was soothing; their alternate dominance and submissiveness, their gentle biting, the pause and sudden pounce, the soft paw on paw, belly on belly. Rather than go uphill, we decided that day to walk along the coastal path, the part that always makes me think of my mother – a magical, open expanse, light breaking in beams through the clouds, the sea beyond silvery grey and endless. Charlie was taking his time behind me, taking in the colours and sights and sounds.

'I want to help you, but I have nothing to give you,' he said, a little dramatically, when he caught up with me. I told him that this wasn't true, that he had given me the two most important things in my life: our daughter and my vocation as a writer.

He pulled off his beanie hat to let the winter sun warm his bald head – 'I need to get some sun on my barnet,' he said, as he always did. And then a line lodged in his brain since schooldays: 'And I shall have some peace there, for peace comes dropping slow...'

A woman with several dogs walked towards us. The dogs stopped to sniff each other, Sunny snatched a dropped tennis ball, they panted and curled around our legs. 'A swirl of dogs,' Charlie said and the woman laughed.

'A swirl. That's exactly the right word,' I said as we walked on.

He smiled, twirled his stick like a baton; Sunny by his side, me, always slightly ahead. And there it was, a memory, even as it was being made, and happiness, however fleeting.

9

'Do you have any hobbies?' a friend of mine from the Civil Service once asked Charlie. He didn't know how to respond, but the childlike formality of this question still makes him giggle. If I had to answer for him now I would say that his favourite hobby is sleep. He's in bed by eight each evening, doesn't get up before ten in the morning and likes at least one nap during the day. He needs more sleep than a toddler, yet often complains of feeling tired. Tired and cold. He wears his beanie hat and thermal socks in bed and keeps the electric blanket on high. His extreme thinness and baldness make him less able to tolerate cold weather and also make him appear more physically unwell than he is.

Often when I arrive at the apartment in the morning it is in darkness and Charlie's still in bed, the duvet pulled tight around his chin. He really looks as if he might be dead. This was how I found my granny when

I was seventeen: she died in her sleep, rigor mortis had set in and though she was gone her arthritic fingers gripped the bedclothes.

Charlie still sometimes pretends to be dead, just as he did to scare his parents when he was a boy, the bed in disarray from a night of fighting demons, his eyes turned heavenward, his tongue lolling out of the side of his mouth. He will stay absolutely still for long enough to frighten me, then he will reach out a thin, cold, blue-veined hand, grab me around the wrist and laugh that he'd fooled me again. And I will feel angry with him for giving me such a shock and at the same time reassured that he is still so much himself.

The range of medicines he has to take to treat his cognitive symptoms and his depression and anxiety contribute to his fatigue. The doctors suggest regular fresh air and exercise to combat tiredness and Charlie complies with this advice daily, as he always has done. He takes Mr Blue out for long beach and hill walks with either me or his favourite carer, Myles – a bright and cheery man, full of chat and interesting facts, who gets about by bike. In an attempt to lift Charlie's mood, he one day suggests that they do up Charlie's old bicycle together – the beautiful American one that he used to cycle along Sandycove seafront to meet me off the train – perhaps Charlie could then go for bike rides around the area on his own. But it is Charlie who realizes, before they have even begun this task, that it is not safe for him to ride a bike any more. Since his diagnosis he has been banned from driving his car. He no longer understands traffic and his spatial awareness has become very poor; he becomes disorientated in any new environment. Even a bike ride together seems too hazardous when they consider it properly. The plan is abandoned, Charlie donates the old bike to the young boy upstairs, and Myles reads to him for an hour instead – a chapter from my second novel – before his afternoon nap. With no possibility of cycling and no news yet of space for Charlie to paint at the Alzheimer's centre, that leaves him only with sleeping, walking, television and visits from friends.

The TV is always on during the day and Charlie sits through *True Crime, Hoarders, Judge Judy* and *Unsolved* on CBS Reality. 'Are you going with that Murgatroyd?' he often asks me, meaning the journalist Donal McIntyre, whom I'd briefly gone out with in my twenties. Charlie has always felt irritated by Donal –

a handsome undercover TV reporter – and gets his surname wrong deliberately. He's seen him most recently on an episode of *Unsolved* where Donal investigates the murder of Michaela McAreavey, killed on her honeymoon in Mauritius. The channel shows repeats of this one episode and Charlie watches it every time, telling me again and again that Murgatroyd is 'bloody useless' as he *still* hasn't solved the murder.

Adverts for Concern with images of starving African children send him searching for a pen and paper so he can take down the details he needs to make a donation, but he can never find these items in time and it's too difficult for him to transcribe the numerals on the screen – and he has no money to transfer. More and more he likes to watch the news. He is horrified by war, ISIS attacks, bombs, explosions, but captivated by them too, he can't get enough of them. I've been feeling the same – when I turn on the radio in the morning I want to hear news of crashes and shootings to reconfirm my belief that life is unremittingly bleak.

*

Living on his own and single for the first time, Charlie becomes bored and lonely. He rarely has visitors; the only people he sees regularly are me, Domino, Mariad and his two paid carers. His childhood friends from the North – Sam, Bill and Hayden – travel down as often as they can and give Domino and me a week of respite every few months by bringing him back with them on the train to Bangor. Pamela, a close friend of Mariad's, visits him whenever she is in Dublin – he goes to bed happier on those days – but he sees no one else. When he first moved here there was a lot of talk from his Dublin friends of visits and of help-ing us out, but none of it ever materialized. Perhaps they are frightened or are unsure of how they should behave around Charlie, or perhaps they aren't visiting because Charlie had never invested enough in these friendships to make any of them feel it was their obli-gation to check in on him, to keep him company, to distract him from his dementia, to see if he needed anything in the shops.

This saddens me. They will all be there at his funeral, with their memories and eulogies, but this is when he needs his friends, during these precious days while he is still lucid, while he is still Charlie. Domino and I receive many phone calls and texts inquiring about him, but having to constantly update absent friends on Charlie's mood and condition does not feel like support; it wears us out.

Because he refused to socialize much with any of my friends in the years we were together, they don't now know him well enough to visit or feel inclined to do so. Occasionally Charlie is invited to a lunch or dinner and he will receive a lot of attention from everyone, possibly because they feel pity for him and guilty that they haven't been in touch. They will often tell me how well he is doing, noting things he remembered in their conversations, or how articulate he is, how well he still looks. Sometimes I will take encouragement from their words, but at other times, when I am feeling vulnerable or sensitive, it sounds accusing: had I exaggerated his illness? Why was I complaining so much – Charlie is excellent company. Had I invented this crisis?

He asked me to marry him last week. I had just poured him a glass of red wine and had begun to 'make' him his tea – two Marks and Spencer jacket potatoes, pre-filled with cheddar cheese, and a rocket salad. I was sitting in front of the gas fire when he got down on one knee, literally. I told him we didn't have the money for a wedding; he sat back on his heels and laughed. Then he told me that he loved me, that he adored me, that if I left him he would walk into the sea.

I hated that I couldn't take his proposal seriously. Not because he is ill and therefore not 'marriage material', but because I wish he had asked me many years ago, before our relationship was broken. And the way he had asked me, half-joking, as if he never expected me to take him seriously.

His spirits, all our spirits, are lifted when Bono and Ali Hewson commission him to create a design for the doors of a lift in their house. Charlie designed an original set of doors for this lift some years ago, so he knows what it will entail, and the project will not only give him something to do, it will give him the promise of some money and, we hope, will increase his confidence and get him back to painting again.

It takes several months to get going, for Charlie to fully understand his brief, to get the precise measurements of the doors, to purchase the wood which he will use as a base on which to work. Domino helps him set up the project in the sitting room of the flat. The room is small and dark and the drawing surface is large: once it has been erected we all have to sidle between the end of the plywood sheet and the fireplace to reach the TV or to put on a CD. To sit down, we have to slide behind the plywood to the sofa. The upstairs neighbour brings a halogen lamp to increase light in the room, Domino buys stamps, finds old poems and images he can use in the design. At first this feels like a solution, and Charlie begins his work.

Domino works alongside him, tentatively to begin with, wanting her dad to take the lead, but when Charlie tries to draw they both know, without saying anything, that he is no longer able to achieve what he wants. He is hesitant and faltering, his hand hovers over the sheet; he is nervous of putting his pencil on the page, of making mistakes. He blames his poor eyes, his floaters, his Specsavers glasses. He is restless and distracted too, stopping every few minutes to blow his nose – 'I need a snotser,' he will say. Or a book or a photograph will catch his attention, and he will sit down on the sofa and try to make sense of it, to match it to his memory. The images he attempts are much less complex than they once were, the patterns more childlike and simple and often quite distorted. He and Domino work for a couple of hours together each day: she closely monitors his mood, discreetly adds letters to words where they are missing, rubs out and redraws or improves his imperfect work and gently suggests that they finish up when she senses he's becoming overwhelmed. For the rest of the time the project remains *in situ* – it took so long to assemble and there is nowhere else for it to go – but it becomes a negative thing, an obstacle and a source of guilt: the largely blank sheet that needs to be filled, a daily reminder to Charlie of all he can no longer do.

Like the objects Charlie has collected throughout his life – the skulls, the knives, the religious iconography, the Kewpie dolls – his art is so much part of his identity that to accept that he is no longer able to draw or paint is another profound loss for all of us. More than the thoughts and ideas he wants to convey, which often dissipate mid-sentence, more than the childhood stories he tries to recall or the bright tales from LA, his work has been his mode of expression. It was his way of dealing with the murder of the boy in Belfast all those years ago, his method of making sense of all he saw in the Troubles, the reason he could hold his head high as he walked down Grafton Street when he returned from America after the bubble had burst. For all this to be gone is too harrowing for Charlie to take in – and yet I think he has been privately worried about something being not right in his mind for many months, perhaps years.

*

When Domino phones to tell me that Charlie has run away again, I'm at my sister's house in Blackrock. My sister doesn't want me to take the call, not because she doesn't want me to talk to Domino, but because she's worried that I'm under too much stress. Domino is always considerate of my free time, so I know it must be some sort of emergency. She's tearful and panicking. She tells me her dad got into a rage while they were working on the project that afternoon and that he ran out of the flat, saying he was going to jump off the top of Killiney Hill. She followed him as he ran up Killiney Hill Road and into an estate near the top. When she caught up with him he threw his hat at her, pulled off his sweater, flung that at her too, then climbed a fence and escaped from her into a field behind the houses.

I phone the police; they dispatch two cars and an ambulance. Domino continues to search for him around Killiney; Mariad travels out from the city centre and goes to wait at Shanganagh Terrace in case he returns there. The thought of him wild-eyed and livid, trying to orientate himself in a world that no longer makes sense, makes all of us panic – but the other emotion I feel is fury towards Charlie – we are doing all we can to help him. Why is he putting all of us through this again? Is he just looking for attention? And then I'm furious with myself for being so selfish and so lacking in empathy.

And when I meet Domino and Mariad at Shankill Police Station that evening – after several hours, Charlie made his way back to Shanganagh Terrace and was met there by the police and ambulance crew – I feel exceptionally angry: with Charlie, with the police for taking him to the station when he has done nothing wrong, with myself.

When I enter the room where Charlie is being held, he leaps out of his chair, goes to the window, grabs the security bars, then whacks them with his fists and roars: 'Get her away from me. She's run off with our child!' The guard restrains him and asks me to leave, says that I am upsetting him. I can still hear him shouting from where I wait in the corridor. Mariad and Domino are huddled together there, their faces creased with concern.

Charlie is being treated as if he is not in his right mind, yet what he is saying is true. I have left him, and I have taken our child, and I am beginning a new life without him. Though we have had the conversation many, many times, it seems that he is only realizing now, on a lucid day, that our relationship is irrevocably altered.

I am mouthy and rude to the police. Domino and Mariad look startled by my pushiness; I'm a little startled by it too. I do not recognize myself, this person so full of aggression and rage. I tell them that Charlie needs to be admitted to hospital as a matter of urgency. They say that he is refusing to go, and that they cannot admit him involuntarily. I tell the police that they must persuade him, that he will take his own life if he isn't admitted, that he will leave our daughter without a dad.

*

The Nipe has her goggles on in the bath, the straw in her mouth is her pretend snorkel, she's watching a Minecraft video on my phone while I delouse her head. We've been here a thousand times – a different bath, a different outbreak, but it's been an almost weekly chore for the last three years. In the same way that mosquitos can't resist her ('I'm just too juicy,' she says), lice like to make a home on her scalp. This is not what I want to do tonight after the drama with Charlie, but her school sent a note home telling all of us to check and treat on the same designated evening.

I drag the metal comb through her hair, but the teeth jam at her tangles and when I tug she screams and shimmies to the far side of the tub. I haul her back, shampoo her hair, then ask her to rinse her head under the water. When she's submerged she thinks it's funny to pretend she can't hear me; tonight this drives me insane. I get soap in her eyes when I try to help her rinse, she moves out of reach again, and I go from calm to furious in seconds, just as my mum always did. I grab hold of her small arm and yank her back towards me.

'Stop it. Stop it. Stop!' I hiss, shaking her arm too vigorously. She doesn't cry; she just looks at me very steadily, and I can see she is scared. I scream into the air, leave the room and slam the door, catching and breaking the leg off a little wooden Pinocchio, a gift from her dad, as I go.

'Mum!'

'No,' I say. 'Don't talk to me. Not another word. Leave me alone.'

I curl up on the window seat in the sitting room and watch a trawler setting out across Killiney Bay to pick up its lobster pots. I recall the way Charlie had looked at me at the police station earlier – with hatred and fear in his eyes. I count to ten, go back to the bathroom.

'Out you get, please,' I say in the stern and weary voice she knows not to disobey. She stands up in the water and raises her arms to be picked up. I lift her out and lower her on to the bath mat. Tonight I won't rock her on my knee or sing 'Mocking Bird' or 'Moon River' as I've done at bath time since she was a baby. She stands shivering in front of me, her hair dripping. I towel her down from where I sit on the closed toilet seat.

'I really miss TV,' she says as we eat dinner. She begins to cry, her small chest heaving at the utter injustice of my banning it for the evening.

I tell her not to mention it again.

'OK. But I'm really, really sorry Mum.'

'Show me you're sorry.' She hates when I say this. More tears and threats.

Before bed she comes close, hugs me, examines my face.

'Mum, can I talk to you in human language not in sorry language?'

'OK, what is it?'

'Why do you never get cross with Dad? And you only get cross with me?' I am trying to think of how to respond to this when she pulls a face at me. 'No offence Mum but you've got green stuff between your teeth.'

I unpick the broccoli with my finger, using her as my mirror, and settle her into my bed. She recites her prayer extra loudly tonight so that I can hear her from where I'm making myself hot milk in the kitchen:

Imagine all the pets in my family cuddled up together, the pets that have passed away before they got to be born, the pets in different countries, the pets that speak differently to other pets. Pets that are loved, pets that are not loved, pets that are weird, pets that are normal, pets that are just special, cuddled up together.

And the humans cuddled up together with the pets, humans that have passed away before they got to be born, the humans that are in

different countries, humans that speak differently to other humans, humans that are loved,
humans that are not loved, humans that are
weird, humans that are special and the humans
that are just normal, cuddled up together with
the pets.

God, please keep me safe and have happy
dreams. Hope everybody else is safe and has
happy dreams. And good days. We'll just have
to see about my days.

God, the thing I'm actually asking you is
please keep me safe and have happy dreams and
that my mum has a good book deal and that my
whole friends and family are safe in their beds
this night.

Then I hear her blow three kisses to God.

Like her father, she often talks in her sleep. Her
sleeping voice is smaller than her daytime one: munch-
kin-like, bright and engaged. Sometimes she will do
maths sums aloud, or she'll sit suddenly upright to
make an important point in an argument she must
have had at school that day, but mostly it's babble and
brief: a few words, a flipping of her pillow, then back

down and she's gone. I read beside her but give up early tonight, because I'm too tired and too addled to take in the words. I slurp my hot milk, meet a lumpy bit of skin that I pick out and trail over the edge of the mug, take another gulp to wash down two Panadol Night and half a Xanax snuck from Charlie's blister pack. The dog pit-pats in and out of the room, unable to settle either.

I wake, terrified. I don't recognize the room; I don't know what time it is. Something catastrophic and unavoidable is about to happen. My sleeping mind understands exactly what it is and that I can do nothing to prevent it. This dreaded thing is familiar; it has been anticipated many times before – but my conscious mind cannot make any sense of it. I am shaking, my stomach cramping. The terrible thing is about to happen, and I can't do a thing to stop it.

10

'Will you mind my knives and guns?' Charlie asks, as he stands and scans his bedroom for other possessions that might be taken from him. These words suggest no violence or danger when he says them, rather they describe items so familiar to me and so precious to Charlie that they are as benign as the childhood teddy bear he picks up next. 'Ach, Ted,' he says quietly as he holds the ancient bear. He examines him, smooths his hand-knitted sweater, adjusts one of his replaced ears. He passes the bear to me, and I lay him on top of a folded pile of clothes in his holdall – tartan pyjamas, warm sweaters, cardigans, two pairs of slippers. I zip it up to help us feel ready, knowing I will have to unzip it again.

I promise to keep his weapons safe while he is gone and pat the space beside me on the bed to encourage him to sit down. He sits, removes his beanie hat, holds it between his knees and runs both his hands along the sides of his head. I rub my hand on his back and feel the hard ridges of his curved and protruding spine. I look at the small blue vein that zigzags along his left temple – its undulations remind me of those toys of sliding beads on wires you find in doctors' waiting rooms. I've always liked its blueness and its detail. Tiny white hairs have sprouted across his pate, as he likes to call it – his razor, that needs to be packed – and there's a purpling scab at the top of his forehead where he whacked himself on an open cupboard door two nights ago.

'I'm dripping from the nose,' he says, on his feet again and at his bedside table, looking for but not finding the toilet roll he keeps there. He has a cough that no pill has cured, a runny nose that cannot be stemmed. I lean over, tug free a piece of paper and give it to him; he wipes his nose and examines the various things that he has assembled on the table and needs to keep careful track of: his wallet, his watch, his phone, half-a-dozen glasses cases – all the inanimate objects that conspire against him daily. Their necessity and elusiveness can make him cry with frustration. He opens one case with a creak – empty – and lets it snap closed again.

Mr Blue is in the room with us, though he does not want to be. His head is bent forward, his snout working at the dusty base of the shut door. He quietly whimpers to be free. The doctor and the public health nurse are confined to the sitting room opposite us. When we left them, Nurse B was sitting forward and uncomfortable on the sofa, Doctor C was standing, eyes fixed on the parquet floor, as he made a phone call. 'No, I *do* like dogs,' he'd said when I'd let him in and had told Charlie to keep hold of Blue's collar; 'I do like dogs, but I am *frightened* of dogs,' he'd explained to me without smiling.

Today, tea and small talk are not needed. This is not a routine visit to run through a list of questions that Charlie can no longer answer – Where do you live? What year is it? What age are you? – or to ask him to sign more forms. He still tries to write his name with speed and flair, as though he were signing autographs, but his hand shakes and the letters miss the line and slope downwards on the page.

Nurse B knocks on the bedroom door. I ease myself out, trying to keep the dog contained, and close the door behind me, leaving Charlie on his own and unable to hear our conversation about him. There's a bed available in the psychiatric unit of a large nearby hospital; they are holding it for Charlie. He still emphatically does not want to go to hospital, but he has run out of stamina and the words required to make a strong counter-argument. The news makes everyone move more swiftly, as though the bed might be taken by someone else if we don't hurry up. Charlie starts moving from room to room too, but he doesn't know what he needs to do, so he returns to the bedroom and sits again on the edge of the bed. Fresh air billows through the flat, doors slam, cars reverse outside, people arrive and leave, everything is in motion. Doctor C and I stand below the listing Parisian lamp, still held together with duct tape. 'How long for?' I ask, expecting days. 'Four to six weeks,' he says.

Charlie shouts for me. 'I can't get my sock on!'

I go in, take it from him, roll it on to his cold, blue-white foot.

'I can't do fucking anything.'

We sit down again together, me with my hand over his shoulder, him with his head bent, crying. I know he is frightened, and I know that when he feels stressed, thinking clearly is hardest for him. I guide his arms through the sleeves of his coat, fasten the buckle on his belt.

The invasion of the home of the unwell person is over. The unwell person is being removed. Blue sees the signs – coat, hat, keys, a final pee – that tell him his master is taking him for a walk. He knows not to jump up, but his tail is wagging so swiftly his whole rear end moves from side to side. He keeps his eyes fixed on Charlie, circles him, paws skittering on the parquet floor. He pushes through the front door ahead of us; 'Jesus, Blue, no!' I shout. I grab him by the collar, too roughly for his age, taking my tiredness and anger out on the dog. I fling him back into the hall and slam the door so hard I can see him cower through the stained-glass window.

*

We hold hands and run up the grey cement steps from the car park to the hospital entrance. 'Remember this, Mum,' my child says, striding over to the hand sanitizer. She rubs foam through her small fingers, watches critically as I do mine, then turns and stamps on the mat to make the automatic doors open. She

195

walks swiftly through, head down, not trusting that they won't slam closed on her. From the safety of the far side she waves her arms at me to hurry up so that we won't be separated.

'I'll be the leader,' she says, letting go of my hand and running ahead. I follow her, warning and apologizing as she negotiates people in wheelchairs, strangers, intimate in pyjamas or lying defenceless on trolleys pushed by whistling porters. She stops at the café to stare at a tiny, jaundiced man, sunk into his bed on wheels beneath a multicoloured crocheted quilt, who is being spoon-fed yoghurt. We saw this same scene at the same time yesterday; this is our third day of visiting. We both like the hospital and its soothing routine. It is warm, clean, busy, safe, interesting. We're excited about seeing Charlie and energized from having had a break from worrying about him. This confinement can't make him better but it will give all of us a rest, he'll get three meals a day, his medi-cation will be monitored and he'll have some social interaction.

My sister is somewhere in this huge building too. She's a nurse specialist in rheumatoid arthritis and, like my late mum, has such a comforting presence that it is enough to know that I could meet her for coffee if I need or want to.

We stop at the shop to buy a choc ice for Charlie. The Nipe holds it and skips ahead again, remembering her way to the Psychiatry of Old Age ward in Elm Mount Unit. It's for people aged sixty-five and over. At exactly sixty-five, Charlie is too old for the other unit, so we turn left at the end of the corridor rather than right to where the younger people are treated.

The Nipe stands on tiptoes to reach the bell to the locked ward. Through the window we can see several men in the sitting room watching TV. Charlie isn't there; he complains that all they watch is football. He hates every sport except snooker and motorbike racing. We find him sitting alone at the far end of the corridor outside the bedrooms, away from everyone.

'I'm all bunged up,' he says as we approach, giving us notice of his flatulence, 'I haven't gone for months.'

'Dada, I have a surprise for you besept it's for us both.'

'Hey, stinky,' he says and bends to cuddle his daughter. 'Wow!' He feigns surprise when she produces the ice-cream from behind her back.

A man in a purple sweater and striped pyjama

bottoms walks towards us and holds out his hand to shake Charlie's.

'Hello, I'm Paul,' he says. Then he turns to me, takes my hand and holds it in both of his. 'Can you get me out of here, love?' he asks in a gentle whisper. Charlie smiles and is polite and squeezes this man's shoulder as we walk on ahead.

'That's Paul,' he says, out of earshot. 'He introduces himself to me every day. They're all called Paul in here. And they all want to get out. They cornered me yesterday, telling me about their great plan to escape.'

'That's Margaret,' he says as we pass another room. 'She's thin and flat as a piece of paper lying there.' I see the old woman beneath a hospital-pink sheet, propped up on a pillow, her yellow hair on end like a newborn chick's feathers. 'Where is he?' she shouts abruptly at a picture on the wall. Charlie says she's looking for her late husband. 'Down in the pub,' she says, answering herself.

Charlie has been given a room to himself with his own bathroom. He is happy about this at first – we all are – but there is no television, and he can no longer read, so there is nothing for him to do. The sketch pad and pencil I left on his bedside locker to encourage

drawing are untouched. Beside them there's the oblig-
atory carton of grapes and an uneaten M&S sandwich.
There are two visitor chairs; on one of them is a stack
of adult nappies. Aside from a liking for chocolate ice-
cream, mint humbugs and Walnut Whips, Charlie no
longer feels hunger and has no interest in or enthusiasm for food.

Charlie and the Nipe sit on his bed. He's leaning
back, cross-legged, his free arm behind his head; she's
upright beside him with her legs curled under her.
The sharing of an ice-cream is a quiet and long-held
ritual between the two of them and Mr Blue, who
gets to lick the stick when all the chocolate is gone.
They pass the ice-cream back and forth to each other
in silence aside from the occasional 'mmmm'. They
are both very focused. 'Hey,' her dad says when she
takes too big a bite, and she gently tells him off when
he drops chocolate on his sweater, helping him to
clean up by retrieving bits and putting them into her
mouth.

'Look at your bake, wee stinky.'

She is momentarily confused by this Northern
term for face. He runs his finger along the side of his
mouth in explanation. She wipes her lips with the

back of her hand and scrambles off the bed. 'Will you play tag with me, Dad?'

'I don't know what that is,' he says, looking at me for help.

'Just chase her,' I say.

'Why you...' he says, lunging at her in mock anger. She screams and runs through the overheated ward.

He likes to say goodbye to us in the living room, where the other men, the TV mafia, he calls them, gaze slack-jawed at the television. I know he is showing us off, lifting his young daughter into his arms and kissing me squarely on the lips. He still has swagger with these men. He is younger, he is cooler, he watches their befuddlement, feels sorry for them and tries to help them. He remembers so much more than they do.

After we have said goodbye, Charlie watches our progression through a series of windows that separate the ward from the rest of the hospital. He shadows us as he walks back to his room. At the first window he pretends to disappear down steps, he springs up for the second, then peers ever so slowly around the third. The Nipe shrieks with excitement and begins to copy him. He finally turns away, walks back into his room and closes the door. She is quiet for a moment and then she takes my hand. 'How about I pretend to be an old lady and you hop like you've only got one leg?' she says, and this is how we leave the hospital that evening: me hopping on one leg, the Nipe bent over, a hand on her lower back and hobbling.

*

For someone who is actively antisocial, Charlie has never been more popular. Many friends visit, perhaps because they now understand how unwell he has become, or perhaps because they feel safer seeing him here, in the controlled environment of a hospital, rather than at home. There is a sense too that Charlie is receding into himself and that the ability to reach him is diminishing with each day.

Unlike the other patients on the ward who some-times don't receive friends or relatives during visiting hours, Charlie always has company. Between the three of us – Domino, Mariad and me – we ensure that every shift is covered and that he always has a visi-tor. In the early weeks of his confinement, his eldest daughter, India, travels from California to visit him. He recognizes her right away; he has always adored her, they share the same quirky sense of humour.

Instead of going to the café in the public hospital, we take him to the brighter, more salubrious one in the nearby private hospital, to make it more of an occasion. Charlie hasn't been here before, and he is restless as soon as we sit down. There are too many people around him, making too much noise, and there's a confusion of food and cutlery and trays on the table in front of him.

India lifts her teacup, deliberately holding her little finger out like a lady – something her dad used to do to make her laugh – then she cuts her egg into tiny pieces with dainty movements of her knife and fork – another of Charlie's foibles. He watches her and remembers and laughs, but then his expression turns vague and his eyes begin to fill. He stands up and tells us that he has to go: 'You don't know what it's like,' he says, struggling to get his arm into his coat, the hospital tag on his too-thin wrist snagging on its sleeve. 'I have to get out of here.'

I bustle into his room each day, bringing with me a rush of cold air and complaints about mundane things that are happening in the outside world – Charlie quite likes it when I moan; he gets cross and frustrated on my behalf – and I listen to his dissatisfaction with his enclosed world. He is bored from being locked into a ward where he has no daily exercise, no visits from consultants ('Where is that cunt of a doctor who put me in here in the first place?'), no changes to his medications, no healthy food and literally nothing to do. When he was first admitted, I asked one of the nurses whether he would be receiving any counselling during his stay. She told me that it isn't offered to patients with Alzheimer's as they won't be able to recall their sessions and it would therefore be of little benefit. I argued that it would help Charlie to talk to someone neutral about his worries and anxieties. Even if it were to give him only temporary relief, some sense of being understood, it would be worthwhile. If it eased his mind for that hour alone, surely it was worth doing. She told me it just wasn't a service they offered to people with dementia.

More and more often, he is asleep when I arrive. I sometimes curl up beside him and wait for him to come round. He likes to look back, to talk about our years together and to retell old stories, but he loses his train of thought very often. As if talking to someone with a stutter, I want to try to encourage the words out – sometimes he wants this help, sometimes it makes him more frustrated still. 'Just leave me be,' he will say, turning his back to me, when I try to prompt or second-guess him. He seems to have no difficulty in recalling things I would rather he had forgotten. He remembers very clearly, for example, that I took all my clothes off on our second date – he had been a little amazed, a little shocked by this level of forwardness, but I had felt immediately comfortable with him and didn't see that it was a big deal. When I left the other evening he asked me to bring him in a *Playboy* magazine the next time I visited. I found one on the top shelf of the newsagent across the road from the hospital but wasn't tall enough to reach it and felt too embarrassed to ask someone to get it down for me. When asked by an old friend of Charlie's what he might appreciate as a gift, this was what I suggested, though Charlie was underwhelmed by the one that he chose, complaining that all the girls still had their underwear on.

A friend of friends – an English woman who practises as a psychic healer – offers to work with Charlie. She brings him a bottle of holy water from Lourdes, Catholic water for an atheist, which he happily accepts and puts on his bedside table. He likes this woman's presence, her softness. He is becoming softer too, as the illness takes hold: less irritated by others, less cynical of their beliefs, more open to their differences. He asks me often about my family – he feels deep regret for how he treated them in the past. He wants to make amends, to say sorry, but worries that he has left it too late and that none of them like him any more.

One afternoon all the children from Shanganagh Terrace come to visit, along with their parents and Val. They are full of stories of Blue – they've been minding him while Charlie has been gone. We'd got into the habit of my taking him out for a walk in the mornings, the children throwing balls for him in the afternoons and Val bringing him upstairs to lie by the fire in his sitting room in the evenings. The children are as sweet and well behaved as ever, but the sheer number of them, the sudden busy-ness of the room, create sensory overload for Charlie. Several people are talking at once; the kids are restless, kicking against the bottom of the bed, heaving themselves up on the radiator so they can see out the window. It's only when I give him a concerned look, only when he makes sense of my expression, that he reacts. This has happened before. It seems that he needs my cue to help him understand what is bothering him. He is suddenly lucid and alert to what he can no longer tolerate. He asks me to ask everyone to please leave right away.

As the weeks in hospital go on, Charlie feels that nothing is being done to help him, and his mood deteriorates. He begins to choose, like a king or president, whom he will see during visiting hours and whom he will send away. One day he refuses to see me, but allows Mariad to sit with him. Another day he asks her to leave and tells the nurses he doesn't want to see his daughters, that he is only happy to see me. He begins to waver between trust and paranoia. Some days he feels certain that we are all lying to him, that it is Domino's fault that he is in hospital because she told the police he was suicidal. He insists that he has never once talked of taking his own life, though he does so often. Some days he switches off his mobile so that we have to phone the ward number instead. When his phone charger is removed from his room by one of the nurses, I ask why this has been done. She tightens an imaginary cord around her neck in explanation, but Charlie is watching and listening to her while the other men line up obediently in the corridor for their tea.

I begin to leave the Nipe at my sister's or with a friend rather than take her to the hospital with me. She doesn't mind this; hospital visits are no longer exciting. When I do bring her – I still want her to see her dad as much as possible so that she remains close to him, but I need the visits to be brief to keep things harmonious between them – she entertains herself on the long walk from the car park to the ward by stepping over the lines or skipping sideways – arms wide, legs wide – her light, agile body moving deftly. Sometimes she will stop me when we are walking so that we can move in time – she'll ask which foot I'm going to start with and will line up hers beside mine and off we'll go in synchrony. Sometimes we'll have a race, but she'll always check what shoes I'm wearing first. She has seen me fall before, has seen my shock and vulnerability, so now she watches me as we run, wanting to win but also needing to keep me safe. 'Not too fast, Mum,' she said to me the other night, putting her arm out to slow me down. 'If you get hurt, I'll be on my own.'

*

The atmosphere on Charlie's ward becomes unstable. Several men there, including him, are volatile, and it's making the staff nervous. A decision is taken to move Charlie out of his single room because there is someone who needs it more, and they feel that he might do better with company. He is moved into a room with George, a former marathon runner now in his eighties, with a large belly and braces. He was admitted because he wasn't able to cope with the knowledge that his wife has terminal brain cancer. She's here in the hospital too, upstairs and dying. The staff allow George out of the ward once a day to go upstairs to visit her. He is warm, kind and lucid and tries to help to keep Charlie calm, but the more agitated Charlie becomes, the more he is sedated. This stay is no longer doing him any good, and we now all want to get him out of here and home. But it is not straightforward: they are reluctant to discharge him until he is stable and he won't be stable until he is told that he can go home. I tell him he needs to be on his best behaviour, he needs to pretend that he feels OK, he needs to stop being aggressive with the staff and to at least try to eat the hospital food.

On the morning Charlie tries to jump out of a

window, George has put on a meditation tape to calm his roommate down. It's a ground-floor window – the drop is only a few feet – so it's more of an attempted escape than an attempt to end his life, but he hits the nurse who tries to stop him. To me this seems a rational act of a lucid man who has been locked in a ward for five weeks without any diversion and nothing to think about aside from what lies ahead of him. He is scared: scared of staff, scared of what's happening to his mind, scared of the future he sees for himself in the bewildered men around him. But the staff of the Elm Mount Ward see this impulsive act as a new symptom of his disease rather than the product of an existing personality trait, and it makes them worry. It's a side to Charlie they had not seen before; if he does something like this here, he could do it again at home. They detain him involuntarily under the Mental Health Act. He is put under twenty-four-hour watch. He is heavily sedated.

In the days that follow, Charlie is moved away from George and back to the isolation of a single room. The curtains are kept drawn, a male nurse sits on guard in the corner. Charlie is immobilized in his bed. He knows now that staying silent is the safest and easiest thing. We begin a long fight to get Charlie discharged, with as much determination as we had five weeks earlier to have him admitted. I ask him one evening if he would like to go home.

'I'll just do what I'm told to do,' he says. 'I'm the fool in the corner.'

11

We're running late and I'm driving too fast.

'Can I *please* have your phone?' the Nipe nags from her car seat behind me. Beside her, in a harness secured to the seat belt, Sunny whines to be free. I slow down at the junction just beyond Finnegan's pub in Dalkey village to allow a few pedestrians to cross. They'd seen my hearse-like car approach at speed and had hurriedly returned to the kerb in case I didn't stop. I watch their anxious faces turn to relief when I gesture with my hand for them to go ahead. As they cross – several teenagers, a mother with a buggy, an elderly man – some of them wave to thank me, others walk on without acknowledgement, and I imagine at that moment what a shock they would get if I were to put my foot on the accelerator and plough headlong in to them. This is how I am thinking now; I resent people whose lives appear to be continuing normally, I resent people with partners, I am jealous of intact families. I observe them with something more than envy: I am baffled and mystified as to how they've made it work when we couldn't.

It's a bright and still Sunday afternoon in November 2015. I travelled with Charlie by train to the North yesterday to deliver him to his oldest and closest friend, Hayden, at Belfast Central station. After his six weeks in hospital, we all felt he needed some fun and a change of scene. I read *Darkness Visible* by William Styron to him on the three-hour journey. People noticed my reading aloud to him, but Charlie didn't mind. Once ashamed of his illness, he now tells anyone he comes into contact with about it. He says he has dementia, he says he is dying, that he won't be here next year.

The book is an account of Styron's descent into depression and his subsequent recovery, and Charlie had read it before, many years earlier. Every so often he would nod in recognition, put on his glasses and use his finger to find where I was in the text. Styron wrote about the potential link between the early loss of a parent and the development of severe depression in adulthood, which made me worry about the Nipe, who will undoubtedly lose her father while she is still very young – though not within the next year as Charlie fatalistically put it.

I couldn't share these thoughts with Charlie because I didn't want to upset him, so I continued reading with a heaviness in my chest. I no longer have great expectations, any expectations, for future relationships. I just want calm and stability for the Nipe and me, and to have something other than silence to look forward to in the evenings. Her father is fading from her, slowly leaving the stage – she no longer likes him to see her in the bath, she takes his hand crossing the road so that she can help him, rather than the other way around, and she has lately begun to call him Charlie instead of Dad. Their relationship is a precious and fragile thing: before he dies I would like there to be someone new, someone to give her piggy-backs – someone happy and strong, with energy, a father figure for her, to making losing her dad a little less painful, to reduce her risk of developing severe depression.

I have relinquished my role of carer for a full week, and today feels like my first day of freedom. I'm going to return to my writing and I've decided to apply for another short residency at Annaghmakerrig within the next month so that I can work more intensely on the book about Charlie and me.

I've arranged to leave the Nipe with her cousins in Blackrock while I meet an old friend for a walk on Sandymount Strand. Somewhere between Dalkey and Dún Laoghaire, Sunny wriggles out of her harness and leaps from the back seat onto my lap, ignoring the Nipe's commands. Standing on my knee, Sunny presses her rear end against the steering wheel and somehow manages to jam the horn. It blares – deafening, alarming – for the next twenty minutes. The Nipe and I scream, Sunny circles, the driver in front gesticulates rudely, people on the street stop and stare. I never use the horn; I find it too aggressive and rude and now, even when I pull over and take the key out of the ignition, I can't make it stop. I career down my sister's road still beeping at everyone – a man trimming his hedge, children on their scooters. Peace is restored when a neighbour gets a screwdriver and removes a fuse, but for a long time afterwards I can hear the horn in my head. It is telling me that I need help. I am in a permanent state of anxiety; I need people to notice that all is not well.

*

'It was just too cold up there,' Charlie says, when he returns from his trip. When I hug him, he begins to cry. He spent yesterday with his older brother, Bill, a former world-champion sailor who lives with his wife in their home town of Bangor. Bill drove him and drove him and drove him all around the country, Charlie says, pointing out restaurants and cafés and things that Charlie had no interest in and no longer any memory of. He saw 'Browner', brother of the late, murdered, Michael Browne, being thrown out of a bar as he and Hayden were walking in. And his sister, whom he had not spoken to for years. He says she was all done up and flouncy. But his dementia was very bad, he says; every time he tried to say something, the words just evaporated. He wanted to go home, he missed me. He missed Mr Blue. He didn't realize he would be away for so long, he didn't understand what was going on.

He has brought back some gifts for the Nipe and has lined them up along the fireplace: a plastic lizard, a black-and-white stuffed dog and a Sylvanian badger – she would no longer have any interest in these things if she saw them in a toyshop, but she knows what she must do; she pretends to be delighted with them. He has gifts for me too: a grey top and a large black platter with a little bird figurine on the side; there was meant to be a second bird, Charlie says, but it fell off somewhere on the journey down and he couldn't find it again.

I remember now that a new carer was due that day. Following Charlie's stay in hospital we have been granted fifteen hours of state-funded care a week – every crisis gives us a little more help.

'I sent her away,' he says without emotion when I ask him how it went. 'She was black as your boot.'

I tell the Nipe to go upstairs. Unusually obedient, she gathers the chocolate bunnies and three white envelopes in her arms – gifts for the children to thank them for taking such good care of Blue in the weeks that Charlie has been gone.

'Jesus, Charlie, what happened? Why didn't you let her in?'

'Hello, are you Charlee?' he says, in a bad Jamaican accent. 'I didn't reply, just closed the door on her face.'

'Oh God, Charlie, why?'

'I specifically said that I didn't want a black woman looking after me. I don't want a Negro in this house.'

I tell him he never said anything of the sort, how outrageous it is, how rude and how upsetting it must have been for that poor woman who was surely apprehensive in the first place, approaching the house of a man she had never met before who suffers from Alzheimer's disease.

'She had hair up to here,' he says, indicating high above his head, as if this justified anything. 'I was scared of her.'

And then he blames me. He says I'd promised to be there to meet her. I tell him I would be meeting her now if he'd actually let her in. She'd arrived early, probably to start off on a good footing on her first day.

I have never known Charlie to be racist. It's true that he had a large collection of golliwogs – one year he decorated the entire Christmas tree with them, and little black dolls often appear in his paintings – but he just saw these as old-fashioned toys. I have never, in the eleven years we have been together, believed that he was genuinely uncomfortable around black people. This isn't Charlie, it's his illness.

We attempt a fight but Charlie is no longer able to argue – he doesn't have the words, the speed, or the verbal armour needed for a good argument; it makes me feel like a bully, shouting at someone who can't defend himself.

I leave the bedroom and put on his tea, still angry with him. I turn on the TV, the electric fire, throw a pizza in the oven, pour both of us a large glass of wine and insist that he gets out of bed to join me.

He follows me in, sits at the kitchen table and tells me about two incidents that happened while he lived in the States. He says he has told me them before, though I can't recall either one. The first was that he was crossing a road in LA when two black men punched him in the face and stomach for no apparent reason. The second was when a black man began masturbating beside him in the cinema one afternoon. Charlie said he'd been too frightened to move so had sat there beside him while this continued and when the man had come he'd put his hand on Charlie's shoulder and had asked him for a tissue. These are the reasons, he says, that he won't allow a black carer into his home.

The wine and my anger gradually soften him and soon he is ashamed of how he's behaved and wants to apologize to the woman.

'Can you hear my ear squeaking?' he asks, out of

the blue. 'Listen, when I chew. Can you not hear it?' I move as close as I can to his ear but I can't hear a thing. Then he asks me, as he does most days, if there is any news of a cure.

*

I'm carrying an overly full bin sack down to my apartment's communal bins the next morning when my phone rings. It's the mental health nurse from Carew House at St Vincent's. At our last meeting with them, shortly after Charlie had been discharged from the Elm Mount Unit and allowed to go home, his consultant at Carew House said he didn't need to see Charlie any more. Charlie was confused and upset by this. Did they not want to see him because he was dying, he asked on the drive home, because there was nothing more that could be done for him? I didn't fully understand why the consultant didn't need to see him again either but assumed it was because the acute crisis was over.

It's raining – the sort of hard rain that stings your face – and very windy. The bin sack is heavy and too full, because I've been too lazy and busy to empty it sooner. The wheelie bins are kept behind a gate at the far end of the car park, and I have to drag the bag down several flights of steps to reach it.

I manage to lug it down with surprising ease as I listen to the nurse. She says they would like to offer me some counselling, that she and her colleagues are concerned that I'm not coping. She says I need to pull away from Charlie – would I be willing to see a psychiatrist to help me manage our relationship better? My sister, brother and close friends say I need to pull away from him too, but I don't see how I can. Who will give Charlie his breakfast and his medicines in the mornings without me there? Who will make his tea each evening? And how can I extract myself without feeling that I am abandoning him or appearing to others not to be doing my duty? I also do not want to pull away, difficult as it all is. I miss him if I don't see him every day, and it's impossible for me not to worry about him when I know that he is unhappy.

I tell her that I do not need to see a counsellor. That I'm managing OK. When I reach the bin, I flip the lid and toss the bin sack in. Lloyd Grossman tomato and basil sauce, well beyond its sell-by date, drips down my shirt, an eggshell cracks and oozes over my shoe. I turn and see an ugly trail of rubbish – rotting kiwis, tampons, a broken glass – all the way back up the stairs to the door of my apartment.

*

Although he was remorseful about the carer he sent away – we asked her to give him a second chance; she understandably refused – Charlie is emphatic in his dislike for his new morning carer. He gets up as early as he can and attempts to make his own breakfast before this man arrives, so that the carer doesn't prepare his food. The man always uses the toilet as soon as he gets there, and Charlie hears no sounds of hand-washing. Then he comes out and puts his hands directly into the muesli, takes out a fistful, empties it into a bowl and gives it to Charlie. And on their walks he yanks leaves from plants, just for the heck of it, carelessly destroying things in which Charlie still sees beauty.

He has also had to adjust to a new district health nurse – the previous one was a gentle, empathetic woman whom Charlie had a soft spot for, but she had recently been awarded Nurse of the Year and had now moved on to higher things.

'Is he sleeping?' the replacement nurse asked me on her first visit, biting into a ginger snap which she'd initially refused, saying she was keeping an eye on her figure.

Charlie was sitting on the sofa beside her, facing her and concentrating hard, hoping he could answer her questions.

'I'm getting these wild hallucinations. They're like crazy LSD trips,' he said, but she didn't respond to him; she looked at me, pen poised, waited for me to translate.

'He's having a lot of bad dreams.'

'And is he eating regular? What's his appetite like, I mean?' I shot a glance at Charlie, answered again for him.

'Is he constipated at all?' I gave her a look I hoped she'd understand. She missed it, rubbed crumbs from her polyester trousers.

'Do you get me? Like, is he having regular bowel movements?'

'Yes, I get you, but Charlie is sitting beside you. Why don't you ask him yourself?'

Charlie had sensed that this was wrong, but he waited for my reaction to confirm his feelings. He got up, went out to the front garden and refused to come back in until she had gone.

*

Today when I leave him, Charlie is slapping a Persian rug off the grass in the front garden – he and his new carer are doing a spring clean of the flat. Despite his own dubious hygiene, the carer seems shocked by how filthy the place is, by how much dog hair there is beneath everything. For months I've been saying that there is nothing we can do for Charlie's cough, but just hoovering the floors once in a while would have been something. Something I could have done, but have failed to do. His cough is always worst in the morning – making him push back from the table on his chair and bend forwards in discomfort. When I hear it, what I hear is: 'You are not doing enough.' Cough, cough, cough.

'Don't be going with men,' he says to me through the open car window as I reverse. I stop, tell him I won't, lean out and kiss him on the forehead. I feel guilty that I am leaving him to go on this trip alone; I feel guilty every time I leave.

*

A strange thing happens when I return to Annagh-makerrig eleven years after meeting Charlie and

Skippy there. Instead of it seeming smaller, run down, less special – as so often happens with memories – it is all grander and more beautiful. The lake is much broader than I remember it and more dramatic, the house is the same ochre yellow, but looks freshly painted and is surrounded by neat hedges and manicured lawns.

I have been given my old room, Lady Guthrie's, and it looks just as it did when I first stayed in it, though the spiral staircase leading up to the old bathroom has gone and there is now an en-suite in one corner of the room. On the bedside table is a hardback book entitled *Annaghmakerrig*. It's a collection of stories and artwork from artists who have stayed there: John Banville, Anne Enright, Colm Tóibín – and me; the first chapter of my debut novel, *With My Lazy Eye*, is reproduced in full.

The sight of the four-poster bed piled high with pillows and cushions makes me think not of romance but of the delicious, rare prospect of a full night's rest without the company of a flatulent labradoodle and a sleep-talking child.

I am here for five days to make a proper start on my new book, and I can think of nothing else; I feel so intensely nostalgic and miss the old Charlie so deeply that I wonder if I will last till Friday. Domino has agreed to move in with him while I am gone, and a friend is minding the Nipe.

I want to call her to say goodnight, but my friend texts to suggest that I leave it for this evening as she seems to be quite happy without me. I tried to get her attention the other evening while she watched cartoons. 'Why don't you go and lie on your bed with a book,' she said to me without turning around. Then she said that she needed some headspace. I sat forward, amused by her use of the phrase. 'Look, Mum,' she said, 'look how close our heads are,' illustrating with her hand the distance between them. 'That's why I need some headspace.' She turned her face back to the TV. And maybe she did, maybe we both did.

When I open the swing door to the kitchen, I can see them all there in my mind: the dangerous writer, the beautiful dancer, the journalist with the flat cap, the poet who spoke only when he was drunk, the grumpy American. But one of them has since died, one has moved to Berlin, the writer never got another book deal and has given up, Charlie will never be back. In real life every face at the table is different, of course, none of them familiar to me. But I am unrecognizable too. Mary from the office remembers Charlie's iguana; she even remembers Skippy's name and that she liked to be stroked under the chin.

I am no longer shy or intimidated by the artists around me. I am one of them now, but tonight I don't have the energy to chat; I listen instead. I look down at my place mat. It's an image of the lake and the boat; I think a set of six would make a good gift for Charlie for Christmas, to remind him of this place – lately he has begun asking how we first met – but the mats are not for sale.

'What *is* that word?' Charlie asked me the other day, looking at the ground as if he might find it there. I knew the word he meant, because we had talked about it every day that week. It was a word he had printed out and given me to use for my first novel.

'Petrichor?' I suggested.

'Petrichor! That's it,' he said, sitting back with relief and crossing his legs. 'You should use that word in your book. Petrichor.' Then he smiled as he recalled that lovely thing: the smell in the air after heavy rainfall.

12

'I've shit myself,' Charlie says, as I put shopping bags down on the kitchen table. 'And I still can't have a bath.' There's no water coming from the hot tap in the bathroom; the one in the kitchen sputters and scalds. There's been a problem with both of these taps since Charlie moved into the flat a year ago; Val and various handymen have come and gone, but the problem persists. Once tolerable, the faultiness of these taps now preoccupies Charlie, and on bad days it can make him despair, saying that he hates his life, that he *has* no life, that he's going to go for a walk and he won't be coming back.

We're two months behind on the rent, because I've run out of money. I had been heavily supplementing Charlie's meagre disability benefit to make the monthly payments, but I can no longer afford to do so. I enter and exit quickly, hoping I won't run into Val, who has never once chased us or complained. He showed such compassion when Charlie was picked up by the police car outside the flat that day, and when I subsequently had to explain to him that his tenant had Alzheimer's disease and to apologize for not having told him before. But Charlie is defensive; he says it's ridiculous that we are paying rent at all for a residence without a working bath. That he hasn't been able to wash for weeks. And he's fed up hearing Val stomping about above him all day and night long.

The flat smells bad this evening, with Charlie's accident and the presence of three dogs – Sunny, who's asleep on Charlie's bed, lame old Lottie, padding up and down the hall, and Blue, who watches us from where he's curled up on the sofa, his eyes sad under greying brows. I've been worried that Charlie has been forgetting to feed him. I suggest that perhaps I or Domino or one of his carers could take over this task. He snaps at me, says he isn't a fool and that he is still capable of feeding his dog. I regret it and apologize to him a little later. 'You're sorry about what dog thing?' he says, and I see that I've got away with it. I sit down beside him, kiss him on the forehead. He picks up a slipper, compares it to the one he's holding in his other hand, then throws it across the floor, not seeing that they are a match.

I go to fill up the kettle to boil water for a bath and I find his soiled underpants soaking in the kitchen sink. I wash and rinse them and when the bath is finally full and warm enough to bathe in, I call Charlie into the bathroom. I'm about to help him undress – he stands with arms outstretched, ready for me to take off his sweater – when Sunny pushes her snout through the opened door. She has Ted, Charlie's precious bear, the one he has asked me to ensure that he is buried with, between her teeth. I yell at her, force her jaw open and tease out the sodden bear. She has ripped off Ted's entire face; there is nothing left but one glazed orange eye.

Charlie holds the savaged bear in his hands, but he doesn't shout at the dog. He just sits there silently, examining the bear that has been with him since he was a baby. The sight of this is too much. Charlie puts his arm around me as I sit down on the bath's edge beside him and fall apart.

This has happened before. At my sister's house last week I'd felt so overwhelmingly sad that I'd had to let myself out of the house and into the back garden, where I'd knelt on the wet grass and howled. I didn't fully understand what was wrong with me – was I still grieving for my mum? For the baby we lost? For Charlie and the long goodbye we were all having to endure? For this illness that is robbing the Nipe of a happy childhood? Or was it the prospect of the future for her and me without Charlie? Something snapped that evening and I could no longer function.

'You stay here. I'll talk to my mum,' the Nipe had said to my sister, when she'd seen that I was outside. She sat on the bottom step of the stairs to put on her runners, struggling a little to tie them.

She stood over me in the garden in the rain, her small hand rubbing my back. 'What's wrong, Mum? Please don't be sad. Please, Mum.' And when she saw that she couldn't comfort me, she began to cry too.

When I tell my doctor how I feel and ask for a short course of Xanax to make me less anxious, he refuses; he says that they're too addictive. I dispense three every day to Charlie. Because he will not get better, because there is only one direction that this illness can go in, despite occasional plateaus, there seems to be no limit to how many mood-lifting, anxiety-easing medicines he is prescribed. The doctors are more concerned with how Domino and I can manage his moods to make our lives easier while minding him. Their main goal is to prevent him from getting too low or too agitated. But because I am still seen as stable, as managing, my doctor refuses to give me either Xanax or antidepressants; he writes me a prescription for some sleeping tablets and beta blockers instead.

'*Mum*, do a thumbs up.' We're in bed; the Nipe's face is too close to mine.

'Shush, I need to sleep.'

I've drunk too much red wine and have just taken a Stilnoct sleeping tablet to get me through the night. I can't lift my hand to give her a thumbs up; every part of me feels too heavy.

'Mum, say I love you.' I try these words – the ones I say to her a dozen times a day. And I think I say them to her, but they must come out wrong. I just want to sleep.

'Mum!'

'What is it? I'm fine, everything's OK. Off to sleep.'

'Mum, one of your eyes is shut. Why is one of your eyes shut, Mum? Mum, Mum, what's wrong, Mum? Mum, why can't you do a thumbs up?'

When I collect her from a play date the next day, she has an impish smile on her face and is angelically obedient when I say it's time to go home. In the car she gives me a little bag – she and her friend had gone to the second-hand shop in Sandycove with four euros from her money box to spend on a toy. Instead of a toy she bought me a pair of dangly silver earrings and a chunky silver bracelet with a huge daisy on the front.

*

Outside the church, parents chatter and pace, arms folded against the cold. We are gathered by the main doors, waiting for them to be opened: internal sounds of the organ tuning up and the small excited voices of children heighten our expectations. A red-faced parishioner finally appears, opens the double doors and bends to bolt them into place. We surge forward into the warmth, keen to get a seat with a good vantage point of the altar. Charlie's just ahead of me in the crowd, but this sudden movement makes him panic – he looks back at me, startled, and feels for my hand, finds it and grabs hold of it.

The vicar, in full robes, greets everyone as we enter. He remembers Charlie's name, shakes his hand.

The organist is poised to the left of the altar, the music teacher crouched below the children as they are ushered into their places, giddy, some of them fretful, needing the loo, seeking out and waving at their parents in the audience. The church is full, even the gallery above us is busy, and the children are difficult to pick out beyond the stuffed pews. The words of their song are hard to decipher, shyness keeping their chins to their chests, and one of the microphones isn't working. Charlie gets restless early on, roots in his pockets for his mint humbugs and tissues.

After several hymns and a play, there is a prize-giving ceremony. There's a big cheer for the Nipe, when her entry for the art competition is announced as the winner. The painting she'd submitted was one that she and her dad had worked on together. Charlie had found an image for her to copy in one of his old Rupert Bear annuals and had guided and advised her as she painted, but when he was in the bathroom, trying to work out how to refill the water glass for the brushes, she made a bold departure from the image and added a big messy rainbow with smiling clouds on either end of it. Charlie was furious when he returned and told her that she had completely ruined it – not recognizing that this originality, going against the rules and painting outside the lines, was the very thing that made her just like him.

We go down to Dalkey village for pizza to celebrate Nipe's achievement. It's early – only seven – and the restaurant is quiet. Charlie doesn't fumble for his glasses any more or try with great effort to make sense of the menu. It's simpler now: I read the menu to myself and order for all of us: margherita pizza for the two of them, followed by ice-cream; a bowl of pasta for me. To drink, apple juice for the Nipe, wine for me and a hot whiskey for her dad.

We move to a different table as soon as we've ordered; the grinding and hissing of the coffee machine are torture to Charlie's ears. And we move again just as our food arrives because we are now too near the kitchen and the clatter of plates being stacked makes Charlie wince and threaten to leave.

I help him locate his knife and fork on the table and place them in his hands; he insists on cutting up his pizza though he finds it very difficult, the prongs of his fork turned upward, his knife the wrong way around. The Nipe sits back in her seat with her pizza in her hand and watches her dad struggle, sees salad slide off his plate, looks at me and back at him.

Our conversation goes in circles, the Nipe inter-rupting continually, me trying to pretend each of Charlie's questions is new.

Charlie: How's your grandmother?

Me: My godmother? She's OK, though she's just
    had a hip replacement...

Nipe: Mum, can I borrow your phone?

Charlie: Fuck. I'm dripping from the nose.
    Where would I find a tissue?

Nipe: Did Dad just say the F-word? Mum, do I
    have to eat my broccoli?

Charlie (getting up, looking for a tissue): Ouch.
    They left some metal in my shoulder where
    they gave me the flu jab.

Me: I don't think they did, Charlie. Maybe it's a
    bruise?

Charlie: Domino's going to get the doctor to
    look at it. Domino's brilliant.

Nipe: Phone, Mum?

Charlie: Any news on the book?

Me: No, still waiting. My agent –

Nipe: Mum? If I don't eat my broccoli can I still have ice-cream?

Me: Try and eat some. Nipe, will you do your Australian accent for Dad?

Nipe: There's a shaaahk in the waw-tah.

All three of us laugh.

Nipe: Want to hear my Indian one?

Charlie: How's the big lad? (This could mean our mutual friend Keith or our old neighbour's autistic son.)

Nipe: Mum?

Me: What is it? Can't you see that your dad and I are talking?

Charlie (putting his head in his hands in exasperation and waiting till his daughter is quiet): Any news on the book?

Me: No, still waiting to hear.

Charlie: How's your grandmother?

Me: Godmother? She's fine, though she's just had a hip replacement...

Nipe, unhappy with her ice-cream flavour: What the weasel in the peasel?

A baby starts to scream at a table nearby.

Charlie: Jesus Christ, I have to get out of here.

When we're getting ready to leave, the Nipe slides off her chair, asks for her dad's hat, and tells him that she wants to put it on his head. She takes the hat – a *Fargo*-like one with fur lining and ear flaps. He leans forward and talks her through how to close the clasp under his chin.

'Do my shoes look angry to you?' Charlie asks on our way out. All three of us look down at his feet. He is wearing brand-new Converse high-tops – the white rubber so bright and the fabric so clean they make me think of Ernie and Bert from *Sesame Street*; of an episode I remember from childhood where Ernie tap dances with pigeons. They are the least angry shoes I've ever seen. We laugh; the Nipe takes her dad's hand, begins to skip beside him. But he stops and asks us to look at them again, he wants us to agree with him. And when we look properly, when we see his feet from his viewpoint, we understand what he means: the way the laces are slanted through the holes makes them look like the furrowed brows of a very angry pair of shoes.

Charlie says he has wanted to say something to me for years, since he met me at Annaghmakerrig. He says he really needs to get it off his chest.

'I've always felt that there is something wrong with your feet. I always have to have a quick check when I see you. I think that they're probably normal, but I just need to be sure.'

We both look down at my feet and back at each other. I look at him bemused. He hugs me and laughs.

'Bye, Dada, I love you!' the Nipe shouts from the back seat when we drop him home. She's agreed to wait in the car while I run in with him, give him his night-time meds and settle him into bed.

Nothing.

'Say I love you,' I whisper to Charlie.

'I love you, darling,' he says, turning to me and putting his arms around my waist.

'No, tell your daughter that you love her.'

'I told her earlier.'

'Well tell her again.'

Silence. Then, irritated: 'I don't understand what you're asking me.'

When I get back in the car: 'Mum? Why wouldn't Dad say he loved me?'

*

Domino spotted me from the window of a café she was in as I walked home through Dalkey village one afternoon last week. She rushed out to catch up with me, said that she was going to ring me, that she had come up with an idea, a solution. She said she'd been giving it a lot of thought and that if it was OK with me, she would like to move in with her dad.

Initially I was unsure: it seemed an extraordinary sacrifice for a woman still in her early twenties, and too much pressure for her to take on single-handed. She assured me that she wanted to do it, that she would apply for Carer's Allowance, and joked that it would save her the cost of years of counselling as it would bring her close to her dad again after feeling quite let down by him as a teenager, when he had separated from her mother. Her only stipulation was that they find somewhere new to move to together – she did not want to live in Shanganagh Terrace.

We agreed that the present arrangement was not sustainable. For her, the long daily drive from Ringsend, where she was living with her mother, was too arduous and expensive. For me, the cost of paying for weekly groceries and rent, of driving each morning to give Charlie his breakfast and again with the

Nipe each night – never knowing what we might find when we got there – and then home in the dark with the Nipe in her pyjamas and too late to bed, was not a routine we could continue indefinitely.

Domino began her search in Dún Laoghaire, only ten minutes from where we live, but found nothing affordable there. After several weeks of hunting she sent me images of a small house in Ringsend. It looked clean and cosy and was a five-minute walk from Mariad's house – she and Charlie still got along extremely well and it would give Domino some comfort to have her mother so close.

Charlie is reluctant when I talk to him about the move.

'Will I be very far away from you?' he asks.

'Not too far – about forty minutes, I'd say. But I will visit as often as I can and I'll call you every day.'

'I've got the two towers there and the beach, and I can walk into the city,' he says, trying to be more positive.

'And you've got the canal.'

This draws a blank – he can't remember it, or visualize it when I try to describe where it is and tell him that we have walked along it together before.

He doesn't know the area well, he will be further away from the Nipe and me, he is not sure about the idea of living with his grown-up daughter – but he knows he has no money and no independence and therefore little choice. I see that he is scared but he tries to be upbeat; I feel a combination of profound relief and profound sadness at the idea of being further away from him, of severing more ties.

Domino uses the money from the lift-door project to secure the new house; the landlord agrees to a year's rent up front. Because of the distress and frustration the project had caused Charlie, it was never mentioned again by any of us after he returned from hospital. Domino rolled it up and took it back to her mother's house and finished it on her own, and she had presented it to the Hewsons a few weeks previously.

The Nipe and I will see Charlie much more infrequently, and we will inevitably become more distant. There will come a day when he won't recognize me or his youngest child, yet he may still know his ex-wife and his two elder daughters. I dread this time, and I will miss him wanting me and depending on me. I dread him no longer remembering anything at all about the crazy, silly, funny, sweet, terrible, heart-breaking and happy things we have been through in our eleven years together.

*

We visit Charlie on his first weekend at the new house. The timing of our visit is not sensible. The Nipe is tired after a sleepover, and I am in very poor form after a night out with a friend who confirmed my suspicion that Charlie's old group of Dublin friends believed that Mariad and Domino exclusively had cared for him since we moved from our home in Bray, and that I had simply abandoned him.

Earlier in the day Nipey had said that she didn't want to go to her dad's new house. Twice on our journey there she'd said that she didn't want him in a new home where she didn't have any friends, like she did at Shanganagh Terrace, and she didn't want him to be so far away from us.

She brightens a little when she sees the *Coronation Street*-style houses and asks if she can cross the narrow, quiet road on her own. 'Left, right, left,' I say as I stand on the pavement and watch her set off.

Inside, she is excited by the little house and how

cosy it is. As we traipse up the stairs behind her, she says she wants to see her bedroom. We explain that there are just two bedrooms – one for her dad, one for Domino – because the house isn't big enough for more.

Back downstairs there is nothing for her to do. She asks for my phone, she wants to be cuddled but keeps changing her mind about who she wants to sit beside. 'It's so unfair,' she says again and again, to herself but aloud. I begin to tell a story; she interrupts. Charlie roars at her to be quiet, and when she isn't he gets out of his seat and stands above her, wags his finger and shouts. She asks him to tickle her; he leaves the room and sits in the toilet at the back of the house in the dark. Domino coaxes him out again and tries to calm him down.

The Nipe begins to cry for her dad and asks again to be tickled. He says no. Then he says that he wants her to leave. She looks at him, confused, and he says if she won't leave he will leave himself.

He storms about the house – up and down the stairs – in search of his coat, hat, whatever. He pushes past Nipe as she sits on the bottom step, crying and asking why he wants her to leave and why he doesn't care about her.

I lift her, screaming and kicking, into my arms and we go out into the street. Her dad passes us and strides down the road, with no notion of where he is or where he is going. The Nipe yells and yells for him with her arms outstretched: 'I want Daddy! Give me Daddy!' she shouts, again and again, as she watches him walk away. She screams the same words, hoarse and snotty, on our car journey home, until I pull over at a garage and she throws up.

13

I buckle the Nipe into her car seat and try to predict any possible need she might have in the next three hours: she's had a wee, she has chocolate, apples, sweets, water, all within easy reach, and baby wipes for when her hands get sticky. The DVD player is fully charged; the musical *Mamma Mia!* loaded and ready to go.

She has a blanket around her knees in case she gets cold and her 'num num', a muslin cloth she's used as a comforter since she was a baby, in her fist. It's now so ragged and discoloured it looks like something from the Famine.

I think of how I travelled when I was her age. Four of us in the back, sometimes five, me curled up on the floor behind the driver's seat, my father insisting on a 'silence competition' for the duration of whatever journey we were on so that he could enjoy his classical music in peace. I would disappear into my dark private world, watching telegraph poles zip by in the fading light, inhaling petrol fumes, my favourite smell, and firewood and fresh manure, as we made our way across Ireland, through villages and fields.

I take the last of four Xanax a friend had given me in a birthday card, and I put one from Charlie's blister pack into his cupped hand. We wash them down with the bottle of water I've wedged between us. Charlie looks set for an Antarctic expedition in his *Fargo* hat, heavy black coat zipped to the neck, gloves and thermal socks under Doc Martens boots. His thighs appear broader than they are because of the long johns he is wearing beneath his jeans. He is sitting upright and absolutely rigid, his hand already clutching the grab handle above his window in preparation for a sudden stop.

We have been staying with old friends in Holywood, near Belfast, for the weekend. It is late November 2016. Charlie's mood has been poor throughout, but he woke in black form this morning and has been talking of suicide since breakfast; at lunch he marched out of the café we were in and we'd had to leave our food unfinished, pay the bill and hurry out onto the street in search of him – it took us twenty minutes to locate him at the far end of the village, snarling and cursing and kicking the kerb.

He'd explained that he hadn't been hungry, and that he didn't understand why we had to eat again when we had already eaten today. The Nipe had annoyed him because she'd refused to answer questions that his friend Sam had asked her. I took this as a criticism of my own failure – we had always argued about discipline, my overly soft style a compensation for Charlie's strictness, unintentionally replicating my own childhood of two parenting extremes. I had been similar to the Nipe as a child: bored by or shy of adults' random questions and observations, ones that they didn't really want or need to know the answers to, ones that bored even them. 'What class are you in at school?' 'What did Santa bring you?' 'Look how tall you've got!'

Charlie and the Nipe had clashed all weekend. 'I want *you* to sit beside me,' he'd said to me any time our daughter was between us, leaning back behind her and stretching out his hand to reach mine.

It's already dark when we set off for Dublin.

'What about my headphones?' the Nipe says as I

put the key in the ignition. I get out of the driver's seat, go around to her door to help her. 'Like this besept not too tightly.' She demonstrates as I lean in to her.

Rain is coming down hard as we travel along the A1 from Holywood to Belfast City, and I'm finding it hard to see. The road is fast and foreign to me, and the feeling that I don't belong on it is forcing me to drive more quickly than I want to; I'm nervous of annoying other drivers, of holding them up, of making a fatal mistake. What Charlie sees in front of him through the rain-splattered window – the blurred headlights of oncoming traffic, endless billboards and street signs, the luminous cat's eyes spiralling along the road before us – is incomprehensible and overwhelming to him, so he doesn't understand how I am managing to navigate. 'Women are a wonder,' he would say in better humour; instead he is silent beside me, aside from an occasional suck of air through his teeth if he thinks I'm too close to the car ahead. I used to do this when getting a lift from my mum, and I only now understand how lethally distracting it is.

He does not trust my driving, though he was the one who taught me. I don't trust it myself, or my night vision which is increasingly poor: my glasses seem smeared with something and I need to replace the windscreen wipers – they're leaving a muddy residue as they try to clear the rain. The speed at which they whoosh and squeak across the glass is adding to my anxiety. The car is temperamental too – it's ten years old and has just failed its repeat road test in spite of the thousand euros I spent on it to ensure it would pass. But I don't want to sell it, as I know it makes Charlie proud to see that I still have a valuable thing that he has given me, something that belonged to him and is of practical use to me.

For the first hour of our journey home we do not talk at all: the only noise is the Nipe behind us singing along to 'Dancing Queen' in that tuneless, oblivious way people do when wearing headphones.

On the motorway there are stretches where street lamps illuminate our way; I breathe out for these bits, but without warning or logic we are plunged into blackness again, the only lights ahead the cars coming in the opposite direction, some of them flashing at me to turn off my blinding full beams. And I have a recurrent sensation that we are drifting to the left and about to collide with the long-distance lorries speeding along in the next lane. I am on high alert, adrenaline pumping, I've been running on anxiety for three days.

'No,' Charlie says, sinking into his seat like a sullen teenager, when I ask him if he enjoyed the trip. I ask then if he's happy to be going home. 'I don't have a home,' he says, that his home had been with me; then he says, apropos of nothing, that people with dementia often take their own lives.

The weekend didn't go to plan. It was tiring for the Nipe and me and utterly disorientating for Charlie, who was permanently confused as to where we were setting off to or coming from. He was quiet and withdrawn throughout; it was impossible to make him smile.

The schedule was too packed, involving too many different people and places. Things that Charlie used to love – walks in Castle Park, by Crawfordsburn Beach, along the old seafront in Bangor – now made him feel too cold and too tired. Pubs were too noisy, restaurants – which he had never seen the point of – intolerable, and other people's homes were mazes of too many doors, toilets that wouldn't flush, handles that refused to turn, bedrooms that kept shifting. His Northern friends' talk was too frenetic, their movements too erratic and sudden. Warm, kind and loyal people, they were doing all they could to try and reach him and distract him and entertain him, not understanding that what is most comforting to him now is the absence of all of these things. A quiet, predictable routine is what he needs. Silence. Warmth. A long hug.

As I drive, their Northern accents and stories, the ones I've listened to again and again over the years that I've known them, still swarm through my head:

'Ach, you see you sitting there, Sam!'

Amanda: bright, loud, energetic, berating her partner Sam, a sleepy eyed intellectual who sits forever in his chair by the fire, a bottle of red wine airing by his feet.

Charlie and I have always loved spending time with this couple – Amanda's energy is infectious, sometimes dizzyingly so, sweeping the Nipe into her arms so impulsively and cuddling and squeezing her with such effusiveness that the Nipe is off-balance and giddy when she puts her back down. Sam loves to tell me stories that he thinks I could use for future books; but it is his and Amanda's retelling of these stories and the way they get along – their body language, their

humour – that is much more interesting to me creatively: 'Just close the curtains on her there, will you,
Charlie?' Sam said quite seriously yesterday morning
at breakfast while Amanda shouted at him through
the window that he'd forgotten to put the bins out.

Evenings in Holywood are spent in the past, in
the company of local characters, many now dead, and
none of whom I'd ever met but whose names conjure
up vivid images in my head: Raymie and Dankie,
Duke and Toot, Mulvenna and The Budgie, The Bear,
O'Malley and Big C, Halse and Kim Lung, Sam and
Sid. Mimi Conway, Cacky Cree. Charlie nods and
smiles with recognition when some of these names
are mentioned, but he can't keep up with the conversations and his expression soon becomes vague. He is
largely quiet in the company of his old friends now
and often closes his eyes, seeming to snooze.

The stories they retell are always wild and humor-
ous; there is never any real talk of the Troubles that
had come brutally to remind sleepy old Bangor it was
not immune to the horrors stalking other parts of the
province. But with Charlie there is always the sense
that Michael Browne, the boy who died in his arms,
is in his thoughts at these times, that it is Michael he

is remembering when he is quiet. Michael's death is a permanent sorrow in Charlie, visible in his eyes, in the lines in his face, in his increasingly stooped shoulders. It is a grief he has carried with him throughout his life, just as Michael's own family have grieved; it's a trauma none of them will ever recover from. Although, unlike so many others from that time and place, Charlie escaped physically unscathed, he too is one of the many victims of the violence in the North. What he witnessed that night in 1974 had lifelong consequences that could never have been foreseen. Without counselling or any way to cope with what he experienced, he has carried it with him and it has shaped him. To imagine Charlie without this murder in his past is to imagine an entirely different man who may have gone on to live a very different life.

On our last evening he woke from his snooze on the sofa and became animated at something his friend Bill said. He sat up and started a sentence so brightly that he had everyone's attention.

'Bill, we must go back to that place...' But he couldn't remember the place he was thinking about. He shook his head, 'It's gone.' We all chipped in with suggestions, like a game of 'I spy':

'Pickie Pool?'

'The garden centre?'

'Ward Park?'

'Stop it, stop.' He put his hands to his ears. 'Please just leave me be.'

I settled him into bed that night while his friends were still downstairs drinking, reminiscing, playing the cheatin'-and-hurtin' songs that Charlie loved. But they sounded subdued, empathizing with their friend's condition and despair, and feeling that they had failed to give him what he'd needed, that he was receding from them.

Charlie's face looked tortoise-like – creased and vulnerable – under the black beanie he was still wearing in bed. He was bundled up unhappily beneath a stack of blankets and duvets at only eight-thirty in the evening. He sat up abruptly and sneezed.

'Why does it always say "Russia"?' he asked me, and as the sound of his sneeze reverberated I understood what he meant – a forceful sneeze does sound like the word *Russia*. He lay back down and curled into a foetal position.

'Will you lie beside me? Please? I promise I won't do anything.' And we lay silent together in the darkness and listened to the singing and strumming travelling up from downstairs.

*

The traffic billboard ahead tells me that journey time to Dublin airport is seven minutes. We are almost home, almost safe. I recognize landmarks, turn on the radio, sit back in my seat.

Charlie asks me if I will come in when I drop him home. I say no, that I will go straight on as it is late and dark and I need to get the Nipe to bed. He says I have to stop being so unfriendly to Domino, that she is a great girl. I chew on my lip; I don't want to go here, it never ends well.

My relationship with Domino has unravelled in the last few months, since the move to Ringsend, really. We were both extremely upset by the disastrous first visit with the Nipe – Domino was annoyed with me for bringing her in the first place when I knew she was tired; she said she'd invested a lot in making the move work and she wanted Charlie to feel calm and settled. But I had felt so angry with Charlie, ill or not, for being cruel to his youngest daughter. She was the most fragile person in this tangle of all our lives, the one we all needed to protect. How could I possibly have predicted that things would go so badly wrong? Since then, relations have deteriorated to the point where we are barely speaking. We are both overwhelmed, exhausted and hurting.

Now that our falling out is upsetting Charlie, Domino and I know we must resolve it. I promise him that I will talk to her, that we will try to make amends. And it is at this moment, on the motorway near Dublin Airport, that Charlie decides he has had enough and that he would like to die. He unbuckles his seat belt, lunges for the door handle – ordinarily so elusive to him – opens the car door, puts one leg out and attempts to tumble into the motorway traffic.

I swerve and stretch over to grab him by the arm. I tell him that if he loves us he won't do this, I tell him it would be a totally selfish act, that he would cause the deaths of not just himself but possibly of many others, I tell him that if he goes ahead, he will ruin my life and his daughter's. He pulls the door shut, Nipey feels the rush of cold air, takes off her headphones. I strap him back in while driving with one hand.

'What dus happened?'

'Nothing, sweetheart, go back to your movie,' I say

sternly. My voice is shaky, my whole body trembling. Please don't hear this, please don't see this. I want to zap her into the world of the musical she's been watching and keep her there.

I hold my left hand firmly over both of Charlie's and drive on with just one hand controlling the wheel for the rest of our journey, in case he attempts to do it again.

14

There are sixty-five cardboard boxes of our belongings in the playroom, stacked from floor to ceiling. They block the window, obscuring all light, and the door is jammed open to accommodate them. I don't know what any of them contain; I can't think of a single item that I have missed or have had to do without in the two years since they were packed up and removed from our old home in Bray.

Everything we'd decided to store had taken up ten units of a warehouse in Wicklow, and I'd gone out twice since the move to send most of it to auction. There were things I'd always wanted to keep – my father's writing desk, an ancient and bockety-legged bookcase that was in the hall of my family home – but I had nowhere to put them in my modern, rented apartment, and I could no longer justify paying to store things we would never use again.

A lot of the bigger items had been taken apart for storage: bed frames with mattresses removed, mirrors off their stands, rugs rolled up as if concealing dead bodies. As the removal men hauled out each item, I put it back together in my mind, restored it exactly as it had once been, and replaced it in its room, before deciding whether it should be sent to Ringsend, Dalkey, a charity shop or to the dump. They slapped tape on each piece and scribbled its destination with felt-tipped pens. There was a small Indian bookcase that Charlie had repaired with his careful hands: it sold for twenty euros; and a chaise longue, with sagging inners, that didn't sell at all but was left out the back of an auction house that was too full to fit it, where mice would get in under the upholstery and gnaw away at the wood. I filled the back of my car with boxes of baby clothes that I'd kept for the baby who didn't make it and then for another future, imaginary baby that at forty-seven I would not now have; I washed them and gave them to a pregnant mum at my daughter's school instead.

'Where's this going?' one of the lads asked, holding up the huge, rusted cross that used to hang on the landing outside Charlie's studio. Another thing I would have to let go: it was far too large for the house in Ringsend. 'And what d'ya want to do with this?' he said, rolling out one of Charlie's nun statues. I could tell that to them these were pointless, valueless items – but Charlie was so proud of all his possessions. There was a story behind each of them that he would retell whenever we had guests. He'd cherished his belongings and had watched wincing as the removal men had inched them over the banisters and through the narrow doorways of our home. He'd intended to keep all of it for our next house and then to leave it all to his daughters after his death.

And yet, since leaving Bray he had never asked about any of his things; he only ever missed his sticks. He had a collection of them – handmade blackthorns, knob sticks, rabbit-handled canes – which he'd kept just inside our front door, in a large stone vase adorned with a lizard. He'd gone through a phase of asking for them regularly while he was living in Shanganagh Terrace; they became one of his unhappy preoccupations. He was worried that they'd been stolen or lost. The removal men spent an afternoon rooting through each of the ten units to locate them and delivered them to him the next day.

Now that all the big items had gone, the units were empty, and we were down to just these last boxes; each containing memories of the life we had lived together. 'Throw them all into the sea,' Charlie said, quite unemotionally, when I told him that the boxes had arrived at my apartment and that they mostly contained things belonging to him. Objects that he had collected over a lifetime, that defined him as much as his art, as much as his matchstick, no longer held any meaning for him.

*

It is February 2017; Charlie is coming to stay the night. The Nipe is sitting on the kitchen table, counting the hours till he will be here. She says she loves having him for sleepovers because he never gets cross any more, and she likes taking care of him and showing him how to do things and that he is the best dad ever because one of her friends' dads never tickles them; another one slaps them sometimes. She is fretting a little that the story we are currently reading together at bedtime, Roald Dahl's *BFG*, might be too confusing for him – but she says she will explain any bits he doesn't understand.

He comes for sleepovers with us most Saturdays, but they don't always go smoothly. One weekend shortly before Christmas, Domino had arranged for him to be driven by taxi to my house and had given the driver detailed instructions. It's a difficult apartment to find and Charlie had got confused, couldn't explain to the driver how to reach me. I'd missed the driver's calls – my house was full of guests for a seasonal family gathering – and when I answered he said Charlie had become agitated, had got out of the car and disappeared. I found him on the steps leading to the apartment; he whacked his head repeatedly on the pebble-dash exterior wall when he saw me, called himself a useless fucker again and again. I brought him into the house, still howling and holding my hand – a cold, dark and distraught figure moving through the perfumed air and straggling tipsy relatives.

And there have been nights when he can't settle; waking half a dozen times saying there was someone at the end of his bed. When he is most symptomatic the Nipe becomes shy and nervous around him, refusing to stay in the room with him unless I am there too. But hot whiskeys always cheer him, as do cheese toasties, warm fires, bubble baths. And no matter how dark his mood, when these things are in place he forgets whatever trauma has befallen him: 'I've never been happier in my life,' he will say in sleepy bliss. His dark moods come much less frequently now; he is calmer, less agitated – but this is a sign that Charlie is fading from us; that the less he fights, the more we are losing him to his illness.

*

'Argh! Right in the balls,' Charlie says when Sunny lunges for him at the front door. Domino is behind him carrying his overnight bag. She has dressed him snugly, as she always does: checked shirt, woolly cardigan, plaid scarf tied tight round his neck. She squeezes past us to give the Nipe a hug and the promise of a sisters' day out soon. She and I hug briefly too; things are much better between us now.

We are no longer novices; we are both tougher these days. We don't flounder any more or cry so easily. We are accustomed to the new Charlie, we know how to manage his moods, what his triggers are, his needs, how to cheer him when he is getting maudlin. We are more proficient, more experienced carers now. The Nipe has adapted her expectations – she doesn't depend on him as other children do on their fathers; and her behaviour – she stays very calm around him now, knows never to scream.

Charlie is happily settled in Ringsend. His Dublin friends have set up a rota on WhatsApp, and they take turns to visit him weekly. I'm not quite sure how this came about, but it is a very welcome development and adds colour to his day. They sit with him on the sofa as his portrait hangs on the wall behind – a second Charlie, watchful and proud – and Mr Blue is curled in the armchair opposite. For his birthday the previous October I'd given him the gift of having his portrait painted by one of his old students in art college, James Hanley, now a portrait artist and Keeper at the Royal Hibernian Academy in Dublin. I commissioned the portrait for some of the same reasons I'd decided to write the book – so that ultimately it would be given to Nipe to remember her father as he was, and for Charlie himself – he loved the happy distraction of sitting for another artist and the very close attention he received. He still loves getting attention. 'Talk about me,' he always says if Domino and I are having a conversation he can no longer follow. 'Notice me,' he'll demand, needy and smiling.

Sometimes his friends take him around to the Old Spot where all the staff know him and he's happy to wander in, even in his slippers, comfortable to be seen as an eccentric, no longer hiding his confusion. He likes his new carers too, has a crush on one of them.

And our child has thrived from having a peaceful and predictable home environment where she can make as much noise as she wants, can have her friends around and can bawl her eyes out if she needs to. Domino's decision to become Charlie's full-time carer has made an enormous positive difference not just to his life, but to mine and to the Nipe's – she is giving her little sister a happy childhood; I will be indebted to her for this all my life.

*

We try to free the first box from its tight stack. I have a go; it won't budge. Then Charlie attempts it, but he is confused about which box we are trying to release. We tug at it again together and it lands on the floor with a thud; from its heaviness I can tell it's full of books. We carry it over to the coffee table and sift quietly through them – dusty and damp works of Shelley, Keats, Byron – and make separate piles on the sofa.

'You have it,' Charlie says for almost everything we unpack. I want him to still be attached to his things, and I feel guilty for taking items that used to hold such meaning for him. I am afraid that I could take advantage of him, that I could leave him with almost nothing, but then I try to be more practical – books are of more use to me now than to Charlie who no longer reads, and his youngest child deserves some belongings of his to be left to her. This feels like a separation of sorts, except we don't argue over anything.

Each box we open contains reminders, fragments from the past that give him glimpses, even if forgotten moments later, of the life that he has lived: photographs of his parents, one of us together in the Lake District, images of long-dead pets, pots and bowls and containers we bought together when we had money, media in formats that he can't play any more – cassette tapes, videos – Christmas cards saved for lists that were never written, brochures from the buying and selling of our home.

'Why did I get all of this?' he asks, a few boxes in. 'I don't need any of these things.'

*

'Wait, I can't get purchase.' I hear the word, I love its old-fashioned sound, but Charlie doesn't say it any more. He starts to, then stops, unable to find it himself. His thumb is trapped beneath the box, its nail already black and dead from closing his bedroom window on it the other day.

He wants to lift this heavy box of books down to the car by himself. He says he can manage it, but even finding where to put his hands is challenging for him – first he raises the box by the flaps, but lowers it again moments later as it doesn't feel secure. He tries again, feeling under pressure to get it right because I am watching him.

He lugs it up and into his arms and walks tentatively forward. I walk ahead of him, wanting him to feel that he can do this himself but knowing that he might not manage. On the steps he is less confident, he inches each foot forward and blindly feels for the next. His legs tremble, then he stumbles, the box falls, the neighbours see, books tumble down the concrete steps.

He wants to try again a little later with a second trip to the car. This time I give him a lighter load to carry, but he is gone too long.

'Charlie, are you OK?' I shout from the front door, unable to see him in the car park below.

'No!' he shouts back at me, sounding in pain. I go out to find him kneeling on the grass, the box upturned, china scattered across the lawn.

'What happened? How did you get here?'

'I don't know. That's what really freaks me out. I can't remember.'

We curl up together in the evening and watch a documentary about polar bears. Wildlife documentaries and Disney movies are the best choices for us now – something that will hold the attention of all three of us. I turn to catch his reaction, reminding myself of my mother, who couldn't concentrate on a TV comedy when anyone else was in the room, as she was so concerned with their enjoyment of it too, their getting the joke. A little later, I read two chapters of what I have been working on to Charlie over a bottle of red wine and a Thai takeaway. I choose the part about our meeting at Annaghmakerrig – he nods and laughs with recognition and is full of superlatives when I finish. He wants to hear more. He lies on the window seat, looks for a few moments out at the sea, then closes his eyes.

'I love you. I miss you every day. You're my favourite person in the world,' he says to me at bedtime. And I feel love for him too. I wish I could get inside his head. I wish I could understand what is happening to him a little more. I'm astounded by his bravery and acceptance and good cheer. He knows what is happening to his mind and he is frightened, yet he is still able to smile and laugh and to see beauty in the world. A walk or a visit from an old friend can make his day. Even a phone call will cheer him up. Watching Charlie is a lesson in how to live life: in the moment and with gratitude for even the smallest joys.

'I think you should get married, Julia.'

'Charlie, that's the last thing on my mind.' I kiss him goodnight on the forehead.

'I have nothing to give you. But not to that Murgatroyd.'

The Nipe stands on the toilet seat to watch herself brushing her teeth and says quietly so that she isn't overheard: 'Mum, I don't mind having a second dad, but can he be a dad that doesn't forget things?'

*

'You can beat the wife, but you can't beat a good cup of tea...' he says at breakfast. I feel him looking at me sidelong, waiting for my reaction. When I smile, his face reddens and his eyes brighten with the thought that there may still be a trace of what we once had.

He is more restless today, reminding me not to forget his medicines, worrying about when Domino might be picking him up. Sunny scrapes her water bowl across the kitchen floor to tell us it needs to be refilled.

'Mum!' the Nipe shouts from her bedroom. 'Can I go on my tablet?'

Charlie is pacing, looking for something in his pockets, then around the room.

'What is it? Your glasses? Your phone?'

'I don't know. Fuck, it's gone.'

'Mum, I'm starving! Can I have chopped-up apple and strawberries with Nutella and a yellow yoghurt?'

'Darling, any idea where my clothes might be?'

'Hang on, Nipe! They're here on the chair, Charlie.'

'You're the best girl in the world. I am happy just to be with you,' he says as I pull his T-shirt over his head.

'Mum, Lucy and Mia and Isabella (her three

imaginary friends) are at the door. Can you dus unlock it please?'

'How is your book going? I'd love to read some of it some day.'

'Can I not take that thing off him?' Charlie asks about Sunny's collar. The Nipe and I had given up correcting him; we'd stopped saying 'she' or 'her' in unison when he referred to the dog as a he. We had learnt to let the small things go. He doesn't understand why she has to wear it and tries to remove it every time he sees her. He has lately taken against other things that I don't remember him having strong feelings about before: apartment blocks, for example. He finds them visually offensive. He says the sight of women wearing tan or flesh-coloured trousers makes him want to boke.

We try to open more boxes, but the job begins to defeat us. It is too much to take on. I've been shifting about things that are hard to dispose of: stained pillows, old duvets and cushions, defunct computers – now wherever I move they're in my way and everyone is trailing after me. Charlie, bewildered: 'Can you show me how to flush again?' The Nipe, demanding: 'Can I've some more apple juice, Mum? Will you put on a cartoon for me?' Sunny, nervy and neurotic, barking at the new and unwelcome items that are altering her environment.

Bored of TV, the Nipe constructs a den in my bedroom – using mildewy cushions from a recently opened box to hold the blanket that makes its roof, stretching from the foot of the bed to below the window ledge. Now to reach my bathroom I have to climb across the bed. I want to be able to walk through my room without obstacles or company. To just go to the toilet on my own.

'Are there still more boxes? Surely not.'

I take him by the hand and lead him to the playroom.

'Good God!' he says and laughs.

We open a box of art books and some of Charlie's old catalogues.

'What is it about? I don't know what it is I was trying to do. It's very minimalist, isn't it? This one is crap.'

'Did I tell you that they've found somewhere for me to paint?' Domino had told me that she and Mariad found a room for Charlie to paint in, in Saint James's hospital. It would be part of a research project into the effects of Alzheimer's disease on the brain. 'Everyone wants me to paint, but I don't know what to paint and I can't see. It's awful when an artist loses his eyes.'

'I learned my good art from Dad,' the Nipe says, now making a card behind us at the table.

This morning the boxes are disappointing and Charlie wants to bin all of it. He empties a full box of his daughter India's things, intended for the boot of the car, into the recycling bin. He wants to help me as I make breakfast. I say he could bring some more empty boxes down to the bin. He does this successfully but can't find his way back to the apartment. He rings my elderly neighbour's bell instead. And she brings him home, cheerful to be helping, her arm hooked under his elbow, still in her slippers and dressing gown.

We are all travelling to California in April for India's wedding. Charlie will walk his eldest daughter down the aisle; the Nipe will be a flower girl. Mariad will design her dress. Charlie says he will do his funny walk – the one he used to do to embarrass them as teenagers, raising one leg high and wobbling, planting it back on the ground where it was before, and finally moving forward with the other one. I say he needs to do a backflip like Willy Wonka when he reaches the altar, so that the guests won't be worried about him.

They practise now in the sitting-room: Charlie first, with a stick in one hand, his wobbly foot out in front of him; the Nipe walks self-consciously behind him, scattering imaginary flowers along the floor.

I find an image of Disneyland on my phone and show it to the Nipe to get her excited about the trip. 'Uhhh, do *they* have to be there?' she says when she sees Mickey and Minnie Mouse waving. This makes us laugh – how could any child object to either of these characters? I think of the ancient Mickey Mouse T-shirt of Charlie's that I wore for her birth.

'Look how beautiful she is,' he says about his daughter, as though seeing her for the first time. Now she is standing on her father's feet, and they are moving about together like they used to do in the old house. Sunny bounces around them, wanting to join in.

Needing a break from their game, Charlie goes to sit down. He misses the sofa and lands hard on the wooden floor. There is a moment of silence. A moment where it could all go bad again, where Charlie could curse or roar or cry, and I could shout and the Nipe would zone out or leave the room. All of us watch him as he sits there on the floor – me, the Nipe, Sunny upright and startled. Charlie looks surprised to find himself there. He begins to laugh. The Nipe giggles, it's infectious, it makes me start too. We stand over him on the floor. His eyes are watering but he smiles up at us. We take an arm each, he takes hold of ours, and we hoist him upright again.

Epilogue

September 2017

'I'm just so happy to be out of hospital,' Charlie says, sitting up in his hospital bed. He has been living back in the Elm Mount Ward for the last four months. He was sectioned for physically attacking his adult daughter and several hospital staff, and has been regularly restrained, sedated by injection and on antipsychotic drugs ever since.

'Who are you?' he asked me yesterday. *Who are you?* The three words I knew I would one day hear – and still, when they came, they hurt and frightened me.

'Julia,' I replied. A blank gaze, no hint of recognition. 'I'm Julia. You love me, apparently.'

'Well, whoever you are, you should probably get going. I need to sleep, and I'm sure you have lots to do.'

'I want to go home. I'm scared,' he says, on days he still knows me. 'I want to see my dog.' He hides Ted, who is missing his right eye now, under his pillow when the ward gets fractious, when the man next door starts screaming for heroin or the French woman cries for her husband. 'I want to go home to 36 Penrose Street,' he says, more wearily as the weeks go by – when it still isn't working, when no one is listening – recalling perfectly the address that had eluded him for the year-and-a-half he lived there with Domino.

When I leave him in the evenings, he follows me cheerfully out until the nurse on duty takes him by the arm. She allows him to stand and watch me go, then encourages him, with reassuring words, back to his bedroom.

Buoyed up by a visit to her dad, who made a gargantuan effort not to make mistakes when he saw her, the Nipe asks if he can come back to live with us when he is cured.

'You know that your dad may not get better, sweetheart,' I say, needing to be more honest with her now that she is eight. 'He might not remember how to walk one day.'

'Well, he can just have a wheelchair then,' she says, furious at me for writing her dad off and for making her cry. 'And we can bring him to the airport in his wheelchair for holidays, and we won't have to queue for anything. We can go straight through.'

We all talk of what we will do when Charlie gets out of hospital – trips to Bangor, revisiting the Lake District, maybe even a weekend in London. Charlie loves these conversations, he often initiates them, but the social worker warns us against actually doing any of these things. The anticipation is enough for Charlie – but the reality could cause another psychotic episode. So we keep on talking to him, keep on getting his hopes up, about things that will never happen.

'Am I dying?' Charlie asks when he hears the words *nursing home*. The doctor renames it a less frightening 'retirement home', and together we tell him how wonderful it will be. How much freedom he will have, how he can go for walks on the beach, have hot whiskeys, even have sleepovers with the Nipe and me. 'Wow!' he says, unable to take it all in. 'Why is everyone being so kind to me?'

'We all like you, Charlie,' the doctor explains. 'We all want you to be happy.'

'I feel like a VIP,' Charlie says, smiling and laughing at us both. 'I'm very excited about this retirement home project, I have to say.'

'Me too,' I tell him, taking his hand as we set off on our nightly walk around the ward. He has put on his khaki parka coat, his black beanie hat and is carrying his stick. He's ready to go.

'The doctor says they have a hut on the sands for me.' Charlie twirls his stick at the thought of this. 'All I need is a new dog.' I tell him that Blue is still his dog, that he is waiting at home for him. 'No, you're wrong. Someone has taken my dog. Never mind, I'll get a new dog.'

'They're going to put me on the sands.' And then I remember the place he is describing – the disused tea rooms on Killiney Beach where he used to paint when he was young. A memory he can still reach.

'And I'll get back to work. It'll be marvellous. I think I'll be happy there.'

Acknowledgements

Thank you to my agent and friend Marianne Gunn O'Connor for turning my life around again.

To my brilliant and lovely new editor, Neil Belton and all the excellent team at Head of Zeus, in particular Georgina Blackwell, Octavia Reeve, Jessie Price, Clare Gordon, Kaz Harrison, Suzanne Sangster and Clémence Jacquinet. And to all at Gill Hess, particularly Declan Heeney and Simon Hess.

To Christine Doran for her exceptional editing skills.

To Rosemary Davidson for believing in this book from the start and for all her excellent input.

To Dr Colm Cooney and Anna Boland at Carew House for their guidance and advice and to Dr Colin Fernandez of St Vincent's Hospital for his constant support.

For early reading and invaluable advice, encouragement and support: Carrie Nathan, Alex Diane,

Acknowledgements

Judy Kelly, Annabelle Comyn, Martina Devlin, Trina Vargo, James Hanley, Eddie Doyle, Niamh Hyland, Joe De Souza, Caroline Osborne, Lenny Abrahamson, Amanda Brady, Naomi Bates, Sam Gibson, Sandra Nolan, Vicki Satlow, Alison Walsh, Sue Leonard and Page Allen.

Special thanks to Annemarie Naughton for giving me a place to write and for getting me through the storm and to Richard Boyle for talking me off that ledge. To Yvonne Moore for such encouraging words when I needed them most. To Val Timon for his big heartedness, empathy and patience and to Sarah Hurding for her magic. To Gillian Comyn for putting me up and for being such an incredible friend, to David, Ciaran and Ray, three of my favourite men, to my wonderful neighbour Angela who always says what I need to hear and to Rosemary Comyn for her endless kindness and faith.

Thanks to my lovely siblings Nick, Alexia, David and Beany. To Mariad, Domino and India for all their kindness and support. To Kip for making everything brighter and thanks, above all, to my precious Ruby Mae for being a never-ending source of joy.